PCOS DIET

LOSING 10%

TO FEEL

100% BETTER

The Whole Foods High-Fiber
Low Sugar Diet To Improve
Insulin Resistance

TAYLOR WATSON

from the Publisher. All additional right reserved.

The information in the following pages is broadly considered to be a truthful and accurate account of facts and as such any inattention, use or misuse of the information in question by the reader will render any resulting actions solely under their purview. There are no scenarios in which the publisher or the original author of this work can be in any fashion deemed liable for any hardship or damages that may befall them after undertaking information described herein.

Additionally, the information in the following pages is intended only for informational purposes and should thus be thought of as universal. As befitting its nature, it is presented without assurance regarding its prolonged validity or interim quality. Trademarks that are mentioned are done without written consent and can in no way be considered an endorsement from the trademark holder.

Table of Contents

PART I

PCOS Diet

PCOS is now a growing problem among women, and in this chapter, we are going to discuss a special diet that is going to help you get past it.

Chapter 1: What Is PCOS?

Quite a lot of you might have come across the term 'PCOS.' Polycystic ovary syndrome or polycystic ovarian syndrome is a very common hormonal disorder that is known to affect women aged 15 to 44 years, i.e., child-bearing years. Reliable studies state that nearly 2.2 to 26.7% of women of the above-mentioned age group suffer from PCOS. This condition affects the hormone level of a woman. Such a condition might affect your fertility. In women, PCOS is the most general cause of infertility. You might skip your menstrual period for such hormone imbalance. Moreover, getting pregnant becomes harder for those women who are going through such health conditions.

Usually, women who suffer from PCOS might face prolonged or infrequent menstrual periods. In some cases, predicting the exact date of periods becomes difficult. If you have PCOS, then the hormones of reproduction are not in balance. Hormones such as progesterone and estrogen that are produced in the ovaries regulate a woman's menstrual cycle. PCOS directly affects the ovaries as well as ovulation. Besides these two hormones, your ovaries even produce male hormones or androgens. Individuals with PCOS have a tendency to produce excessive amounts of male hormones. Many tiny sacs filled with fluids called cysts tend to develop in the ovaries of some women having PCOS. But, not everyone who is suffering from this syndrome has multiple cysts in their ovaries.

Polycystic ovary syndrome also causes the growth of unwanted facial and body hair. Excess androgen secretion even causes acne as well as hair loss, which might further lead to baldness of male pattern. Your skin might become oilier and lead to breakouts on specific areas like the chest, upper back, and face. Numerous reports state that approximately 80% of those women suffering from PCOS are either obese or overweight. Obesity worsens the complications related to this disorder. Heavier bleeding than usual is also another common symptom of this syndrome. Hormonal changes or imbalance also trigger headaches in many women. Mood swings or frequent mood changes are also a sign of the polycystic ovarian syndrome. In some instances, skin gets darkened, or dark patches can be seen under the breasts. These patches can also appear on the neck region, and also in the armpit.

Not only does this hormonal condition affects your fertility, but it also increases the risk of various health problems such as high blood pressure, heart disease, stroke, type 2 diabetes, endometrial cancer, etc. Various other complications include anxiety, depression, sleep apnea, eating disorders, gestational diabetes, non-alcoholic steatohepatitis, etc. An interesting fact is that the maximum number of women don't even know that they have PCOS. A study stated that nearly 70% of women having PCOS have not yet been diagnosed.

The treatment of PCOS varies from person to person, depending on the symptoms and other health complications. Once it is diagnosed, its treatment begins with changes in lifestyle such as regular exercise, prescribed diet plan, weight loss, etc. If a nutritious diet is combined with daily workout, then it is highly beneficial. For those who are overweight, shedding just 5-10% of extra pounds might prove helpful in improving the other symptoms.

Chapter 2: Vegetarian Recipes

Read on to find out some delicious recipes that you can include in your PCOS diet.

Breakfast Yogurt Parfait
Total Prep & Cooking Time: 10 minutes

Yields: One glass

Nutrition Facts: Calories: 238 | Carbs: 10g | Protein: 14g | Fat: 17g | Fiber: 3g

Ingredients:

- Two tbsps. of mixed nuts (the nuts should be raw and chopped into pieces)
- One yogurt (two good from peach or strawberry)
- A quarter cup of berries (fresh)

Method:

1. Take a bowl and form layers of chopped nuts and then the second layer of berries and the third layer with yogurt. You can add fixings into the cup of yogurt.

2. Enjoy the yogurt parfait immediately.

Notes: If you are using toasted nuts, you can brush them with few drops of avocado oil and then season with some salt and sweetener. Toss the ingredients well to incorporate and then bake for eight minutes at a temperature of 325 degrees F.

Banana Pancakes

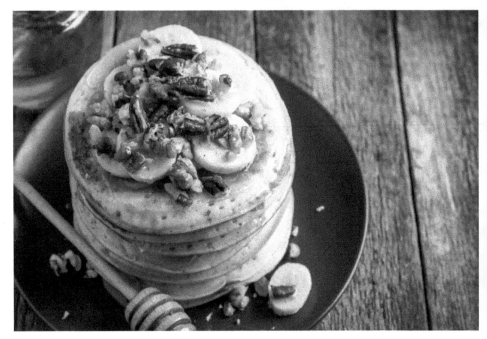

Total Prep & Cooking Time: 15 minutes

Yields: Two servings

Nutrition facts: Calories: 124 | Carbs: 13.8g | Protein: 6.9g | Fat: 4.9g | Fiber: 1.5g

Ingredients:

- One medium-sized banana
- Two eggs (large-sized)

Method:

1. Process the banana and the eggs in a blender to form a smooth puree.

2. Place a skillet over a medium flame and pour one to two drops of oil. For each pancake, you will require only two tablespoons of the egg-banana batter. With this calculation, you can put about four mounds of the dough into the skillet—Cook the pancakes for four minutes, allowing the edges to brown.

3. Flip the pancakes and cook for about two minutes again. Transfer to a serving plate. Repeat the same procedure with the remaining batter.

4. Serve and enjoy the delicious banana pancakes.

Notes: *You can coat the skillet with oil using a piece of a paper towel. Crumble the paper towel and slowly dab on the bottom of the skillet.*

Mushroom and Asparagus Frittata

Total Prep & Cooking Time: 45 minutes

Yields: Eight servings

Nutrition Facts: Calories: 130 | carbs: 5g | Protein: 9g | Fat: 8g | Fiber: 1g

Ingredients:

- Eight eggs (large-sized)
- Two tbsps. of lemon juice
- A quarter tsp. of pepper
- Eight oz. of asparagus spears (frozen and thawed)
- Half a cup each of
- Pepper, green or red (chopped finely)
- Ricotta cheese (whole-milk)
- Half a tsp. of salt
- One tbsp. of olive oil
- One large-sized onion (thinly sliced and halved)
- A quarter cup of sliced mushrooms (baby Portobello)

Method:

1. Set the oven at a temperature of 350 degrees F.

2. Take a bowl and add the cheese, pepper, juice, egg, and salt. Whisk all the ingredients properly.

3. Place a ten-inch skillet on the oven and turn the flame to moderate heat. The skillet must be ovenproof. To the skillet, add the pepper, asparagus, mushrooms, and onion. Cook for eight minutes until the pepper and onion are tender.

4. First, you will have to remove the skillet from the heat. Then you can remove the asparagus from the skillet. Reserve eight spears of the asparagus and cut the rest into the size of two inches. Return the sliced asparagus into the skillet and put the skillet back on the oven. Stir in the egg mixture. Arrange the reserved spears of asparagus on the egg mixture so that it looks like wheel spokes.

5. Bake the mixture for twenty-five minutes. Let it stand for five minutes.

6. Cut the preparation into wedges.

Strawberry Salad

Total Prep & Cooking Time: 30 minutes

Yields: Ten servings

Nutrition Facts: Calories: 110 | Carbs: 13g | Protein: 2g | Fat: 6g | Fiber: 2g

Ingredients:

- A quarter cup each of
  - Sugar
  - Mayonnaise
- One bunch of torn romaine (approximately eight cups)
- Two cups of strawberries (fresh and halved)
- One small-sized onion, cut into half and thinly sliced
- One tbsp. each of
  - Two percent milk
  - Sour cream
- One and a half tsps. of poppy seeds
- A one-third cup of almonds (silvered)
- Two tbsps. of sugar
- Two and a quarter tsps. of vinegar (cider)

Method:

1. Place a small yet heavy skillet over moderate flame. To the skillet, add the sugar and cook for about ten minutes until it melts into a caramel-colored substance. Stir in the almonds until they get coated with the

melted sugar. Transfer the content to a foil and spread them evenly to cool.

2. Take a bowl and add strawberries, romaine, and onion to it. Whisk the contents required for the dressing and toss in the salad. Break the almonds into pieces and then spread them over the salad in the bowl.

3. Serve them immediately.

Low Carb Green Smoothie

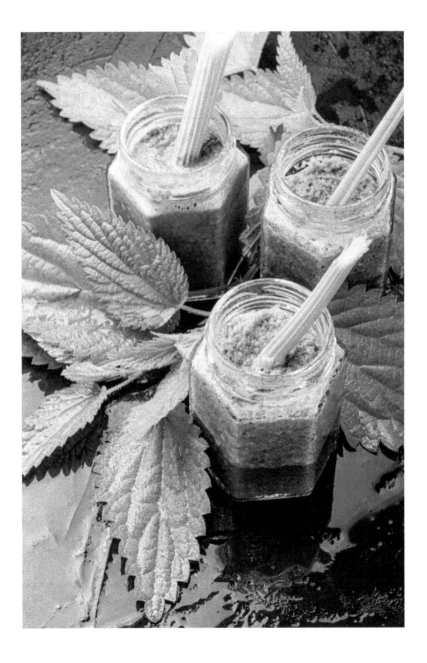

Total Prep & Cooking Time: 5 minutes

Yields: Two glasses of smoothie

Nutrition Facts: Calories: 168 | Carbs: 4.8g | Protein: 6g | Fat: 4g | Fiber: 7g

Ingredients:

- One medium-sized avocado (pitted and peeled)
- One and a half cups of coconut milk (unsweetened)
- One tablespoon each of
  o Powdered peanut butter
  o Lemon juice (freshly squeezed)
- One cup of spinach
- One spoonful of protein powder (vanilla flavored and sugar-free)

Method:

1. You will require a blender for preparing this smoothie. Add all the ingredients to it and process it for about thirty seconds. It will form a smooth puree.

2. You can taste the puree and adjust the taste by adding any component you think is less.

3. Pour in two tall glasses and enjoy.

Peanut Butter Balls

Total Prep & Cooking Time: 20 minutes

Yields: Eighteen balls

Nutrition Facts: Calories: 194 | Carbs: 7g | Protein: 7g | Fat: 17g | Fiber: 3g

Ingredients:

- One cup each of
  - Peanuts (chopped finely and salted)
  - Sweetener (powdered)
  - Peanut butter
- Chocolate chips (eight ounces)

Method:

1. Combine the sweetener, chopped peanuts, and the peanut butter to form a dough. Make eighteen small and round balls with the dough. Take a baking sheet and line it with wax paper.

2. Arrange the balls on the sheet in rows.

3. Insert chocolate chips in the microwave to melt them.

4. Dip the peanut balls in chocolate one by one and return them to the sheet.

5. Place the balls inside the refrigerator until the chocolate completely sets.

Low Carb Cheesecake

Total Prep & Cooking Time: 1 hour 10 minutes

Yields: Twelve cheesecakes

Nutrition Facts: Calories: 600 | Carbs: 7g | Protein: 14g | Fat: 54g | Fiber: 2g

Ingredients:

For preparing the crust,

- One and a half cups of almond flour
- One tsp. of cinnamon
- A quarter cup of sweetener (powdered)
- Six tbsps. of melted butter

For preparing the filling,

- Eight oz. of cream cheese (full-fat), approximately six packages
- Five large-sized eggs kept at room temperature
- One tbsp. of vanilla extract
- Two cups of sweetener (powdered)
- Eight oz. of sour cream (at room temperature)

Method:

1. Set the temperature of the oven at 325 degrees F. Place the rack at the center of the oven.

2. Take a medium-sized bowl and add the ingredients for preparing the crust as listed above. Add butter to the bowl. Combine them well.

3. For making these cheesecakes, you will require a pan of dimension 10-inch x 4-inch. Pour crust mixture into the pan and press the mixture to

the pan's bottom with a flattened cup. Put mixture into the refrigerator for about twenty minutes.

4. Take a small bowl and then pour the cream cheese into it. Beat the cream with a hand mixer into a fluffy mixture with a light consistency.

5. Add sweetener (one-third) at first and continue beating with the hand mixer.

6. To the mixture, add eggs and then beat until the mixture becomes completely incorporated.

7. Finally, add in vanilla and sour cream and combine well.

8. Fill the crust with the cheesecake mixture and pour some of it on the outer surface as well. Bake the dough for about fifty minutes. The cake should have a jiggly center, and the upper part should be opaque.

9. Turn off the oven but allow the cheesecake to stay in there for thirty minutes.

10. Take out the pan and insert a knife in the cake to check if the cake stick or not. Leave the cake for one hour on the countertop.

11. Cover the pan with a plastic wrapper and then refrigerate for eight hours.

12. After the said time, remove the cake from the pan, slice it into twelve pieces, and decorate the top and serve.

Tropical Smoothie Bowl

Total Prep & Cooking Time: 5 minutes

Yields: 2 servings

Nutrition Facts: Calories: 180 | Carbs: 43g | Protein: 3g | Fat: 2g | Fiber: 5g

Ingredients:

- One cup each of
  - Almond milk
  - Frozen pineapple chunks
  - Frozen mango chunks
- One frozen banana, sliced

Method:

1. Add the pineapple, mango, and banana in a blender along with the almond milk and pulse them together for a few minutes, stopping and occasionally stirring until it gets smooth but still thick. You can add some more liquid if required.

2. Pour the smoothie equally into two separate bowls. Add any desired topping and serve cold.

Chapter 3: Non-Vegetarian Recipes

Broccoli and Bacon Egg Burrito

Total Prep & Cooking Time: 20 minutes

Yields: One serving

Nutrition facts: Calories: 259 | Carbs: 9.8g | Protein: 15.4g | Fat: 5.9g | Fiber: 3.3g

Ingredients:

- One slice of bacon
- A quarter cup of tomato (chopped)
- One tbsp. of milk (reduced-fat)
- One cup of broccoli (chopped)
- One egg (large)
- One scallion (chopped)
- One tsp. of canola or avocado oil
- One-eighth tsp. each of
  - Pepper (ground)
  - Salt
- Two tbsps. of cheddar cheese (sharp and shredded)

Method:

1. Cook the bacon for six minutes in a medium-sized skillet, putting the flame to moderate heat. Flip them twice while cooking to give them a crisp. Remove bacon to another plate that is lined with a paper towel.

2. Maintaining the temperature, put the broccoli pieces to the skillet, and then cook. Stir them for three minutes until they become soft. Add the chopped tomatoes and stir everything. Transfer to a bowl and keep aside.

3. In the meantime, take a bowl and place the egg, scallion, pepper, milk, and salt. Whisk them properly. Wash the skillet after cooking the vegetables and oil to it. Turn the flame to moderate heat and then add egg mixture to the boiling oil. Tilt the pan right and left to allow the mix to make a coating at the bottom and then cook the mixture for about two minutes without disturbing it.

4. Flip the egg mixture with a spatula (made of silicone, and it should be thin and full). Cook the mixture with sprinkled cheese for a minute and then allow the preparation to set completely.

5. Transfer to a serving plate. Stuff the lower part of the tortilla with broccoli mixture and the upper part with the bacon. Roll the preparation to form a burrito and enjoy it.

Smoked Salmon and Avocado Omelet

Total Prep & Cooking Time: 10 minutes

Yields: One serving

Nutrition Facts: Calories: 323 | Carbs: 5.3g | Protein: 19g | Fat: 5.5g | Fiber: 3.4g

Ingredients:

- Two eggs (large-sized)
- To taste: Salt
- A quarter-sized avocado (chopped)
- One tbsp. of fresh basil (chopped)
- One tsp. of milk (low-fat)
- One and a half tsp. of olive oil (extra-virgin, divided)
- One oz. of salmon (smoked)

Method:

1. Take a bowl and then beat the eggs into it. Add the milk and sprinkle salt to it. Whisk them properly.

2. Place a skillet (non-stick) on the oven, putting the flame to moderate heat. Add one tsp. of oil to the skillet and then add the egg mixture. Cook the content so that they set with a slightly runny center. It will take you two minutes and not more.

3. Flip the omelet and cook this side for thirty seconds to place.

4. Transfer the preparation to a serving plate and top it with salmon, basil, and avocado. Drizzle the omelet with the remaining oil to enhance the taste.

BLT Chicken Salad

Total prep & Cooking Time: 20 minutes

Yields: Eight servings

Nutrition Facts: Calories: 281 | Carbs: 5g | Protein: 23g | Fat: 19g | Fiber: 2g

Ingredients:

- Half a cup of mayonnaise
- Two tbsps. of onion (finely chopped)
- A quarter tsp. of pepper
- Two large-sized tomatoes (chopped finely)
- One and a half lb. of chicken breasts, skinless and boneless (you must cook the chicken and cut it into small cubes)
- Two large-sized eggs, hard-boiled (slice them into halves)
- Three to four tbsps. of barbeque sauce
- One tbsp. of lemon juice
- Eight cups of salad greens (you must tear the leaves into small pieces)
- Ten strips of bacon (crumbled and cooked)

Method:

1. Take a small-sized bowl. To it, add the mayonnaise, chopped onion, pepper, sauce, and juice. Combine the mixture properly to incorporate the ingredients. Cover the bowl with a lid and keep it inside the refrigerator. Allow it to stay there until the time of serving.

2. Take another bowl, this time a large one. Place the salad greens in it. Spread the chicken cubes, bacon, and tomatoes on top. Garnish the bowl content with egg slices. Take out the dressing and drizzle it over the bowl.

3. Serve and enjoy!

Black Beans and Chicken Chili

Total Prep & Cooking Time: 35 minutes

Yields: Ten servings

Nutrition Facts: Calories: 236 | Carbs: 21g | Protein: 22g | Fat: 6g | Fiber: 6g

Ingredients:

- One three-fourth lb. of chicken breasts (skinless and boneless, cut into cubes)
- One large-sized onion (finely chopped)
- Four oz. of green chilies (chopped)
- Two tbsps. of chili powder
- One tsp. of coriander (ground)
- Twenty-eight oz. of sliced tomatoes (Italian and stewed)
- One cup of water
- Two medium-sized red peppers (sweet and chopped)
- Three tbsps. of olive oil
- Four cloves of garlic (diced)
- Two tsps. of cumin (ground)
- Two cans of drained and rinsed black beans
- One cup of beer or chicken broth

Method:

1. Pour few drops of oil in the Dutch oven. To the boiling oil, add the pepper, onions, and chicken. Cook until the chicken becomes brown and the onion becomes translucent. It will probably take you five minutes.

2. To the cooked chicken, add the garlic, cumin, coriander, chilies, and chili powder—Cook the whole preparation for an additional minute. Stir in tomatoes, half cup of water, beans, and the chicken broth. Cook until the water starts to boil and then reduce heat and then simmer. Stir occasionally for fifteen minutes. You may add some water if you like to have a watery consistency.

Cucumber Salmon Panzanella

Total Prep & Cooking Time: 20 minutes

Yields: Four servings

Nutrition Facts: Calories: 320 | Carbs: 13.8g | Protein: 26.4g | Fat: 2.8g | Fiber: 4.1g

Ingredients:

- Eight ounces of torn bread (country bread)
- Black pepper
- Three tablespoons of vinegar (red wine)
- Salt
- Two tablespoons of olive oil
- Four cucumbers (Persian)
- One teaspoon of caraway seeds
- One small-sized fennel bulb (chopped)
- Roasted salmon
- A quarter red onion, chopped
- One cup of arugula

Method:

1. Set the temperature of the oven at 425 degrees F.

2. Take a baking sheet (rimmed one is preferable). Add the olive oil, salt, pepper, and bread to the sheet and toss them well. Toast the sheet contents for ten minutes until browned and then set aside to cool.

3. Cut the cucumbers into half and then cut them crosswise with a knife.

4. Take a bowl and add red wine, caraway seeds, olive oil, and vinegar to it. Whisk them and then add the fennel bulb, cucumbers, red onion, and arugula to it. Stir well to combine.

5. Transfer to serving plates and top with flaked and roasted salmon and bread.

Rosemary-Lemon Chicken

Total Prep & Cooking Time: 55 minutes

Yields: Four servings

Nutrition facts: Calories: 289 | Carbs: 12g | Protein: 30g | Fat: 14g | Fiber: 4g

Ingredients:

- Two tablespoons of flat-leaf and fresh parsley (chopped)
- One large clove of garlic (minced)
- Three tablespoons of olive oil (extra-virgin)
- Black pepper (freshly ground)
- Two and a half pounds of chicken breasts (skin-on and bone-in)
- One onion, red (sliced into wedges of half-inch)
- One thinly sliced lemon
- One pound of broccoli
- Half teaspoon of red pepper (crushed)
- Kosher salt
- Two teaspoons of Dijon mustard
- One and a half tablespoons of rosemary (fresh and finely chopped)

Method:

1. Keep the oven preheated at a temperature of 425 degrees F.

2. Combine the rosemary, Dijon, garlic, one tbsp. of oil, and parsley in a pot. Season them with pepper and salt. Mix them well.

3. Line the chicken (underneath its skin) with the rosemary mixture and the lemon wedges (approximately eight). Rub the chicken surface with the rest of the rosemary mixture. Bake the rosemary-coated chicken for twenty-two minutes on a baking sheet.

4. In the meantime, take a bowl and add broccoli, red pepper, lemon wedges, two tbsp. of oil and onion to it. Sprinkle with pepper and salt. Toss them well.

5. Take the baking sheet out of the oven and arrange the chicken with the tossed vegetables all around. Again bake it for fourteen minutes.

6. Serve them on a plate and top with red pepper.

Zucchini Noodles and Turkey Meatballs

Total Prep & Cooking Time: 30 minutes

Yields: Four servings

Nutrition Facts: Calories: 526 | Crabs: 27g | Protein: 39g | Fat: 30g | Fiber: 6g

Ingredients:

- One pound of turkey (ground)
- One large-sized egg
- One and a half-ounce of grated parmesan cheese
- Kosher salt
- Two tablespoons of olive oil (extra-virgin)
- Four medium-sized zucchinis (sliced into noodle-like pieces)
- Black pepper (freshly ground)
- Twenty-five ounces of marinara sauce
- Four ounces of grated provolone cheese
- Two cloves of garlic (minced)
- A quarter cup of breadcrumbs (seasoned and dried)
- Three tablespoons of parsley (flat-leaf and fresh)

Method:

1. Add the breadcrumbs, parmesan, half tsp. each of pepper and salt, one clove of garlic, egg, turkey, and parsley in a bowl. Combine well and form twelve meatballs.

2. Heat one tbsp. of oil over a moderate flame in a skillet. Drop meatballs and then cook them, occasionally stirring for six minutes until browned. Reduce flame and add the marinara to the meatballs. Stir them occasionally to cook the meatballs thoroughly and thicken the sauce. You can cook for sixteen minutes or so. After they are done, transfer to another plate.

3. Add oil to the skillet keeping the flame to moderate heat. Then add the rest of the garlic pieces and the zucchini to the oil. Cook them for three minutes until the garlic is tenderized—season with pepper and salt.

4. Heat a grill over a high flame, keeping the rack on top. Sprinkle the meatballs with provolone and then place the balls over the rack. Broil for four minutes until browned.

5. Serve the meatballs with topped zucchini noodles and parmesan.

Cajun Shrimp Caesar Salad

Total Prep & Cooking Time: 15 minutes

Yields: Four servings

Nutrition Facts: Calories: 434 | Carbs: 12.7g | Protein: 29.5g | Fat: 30.6g | Fiber: 6.3g

Ingredients:

- Half a cup of salad dressing (Caesar)
- One tablespoon of Cajun seasoning
- Eight cups of romaine lettuce (finely chopped)
- Six tablespoons of shredded parmesan cheese
- One pound of shrimp (patted dry, peeled, and deveined)
- Two tablespoons of olive oil
- Two cups of diced Roma tomatoes

Method:

1. For the Caesar dressing- Combine one and a quarter cups of mayonnaise, two tablespoons each of Worcestershire sauce, lemon juice, and anchovy paste, six tablespoons of olive oil, salt, and pepper. Whisk them together to a small dough. Set the dressing aside.

2. Pour the Cajun seasoning in a bowl and add the shrimp pieces to it. Toss well to coat the shrimp with the seasoning.

3. Pour olive oil in a skillet and heat over moderate flame. Pour the Cajun-seasoned shrimp in the skillet. Broil for one minute until they are browned. Flip and then cook for two minutes.

4. Take a large-sized bowl and add the romaine lettuce to it along with tomatoes, Caesar dressing, and the parmesan cheese. Divide the entire thing between two dishes and then top with Cajun-coated shrimp.

Egg, Sausage, and Cheese Bites

Total Prep & Cooking Time: 35 minutes

Yields: Thirty-two bites

Nutrition Facts: Calories: 79 | Carbs: 1.2g | Protein: 5g | Fat: 5.9g | Fiber: 0.5g

Ingredients:

- One lb. of cooked breakfast sausage (drained and cooked)
- Three beaten eggs
- One-third cup of coconut flour
- Four oz. of softened cream cheese
- One cup of cheddar cheese (shredded)
- Half tsp. of baking powder

Method:

1. Set the oven at a temperature of 350 degrees F and keep it preheated.

2. Place a pan on the oven and put the sausage in it. Cook the breakfast sausage and drain the excess water from it. Remove it from the pan and set aside to cool slightly.

3. Take a bowl and place the cooled down sausage. Then add the cheddar cheese to the bowl. Combine them thoroughly until all the cheese clumps of cream vanish.

4. Make sure the sausage is cooled down completely before moving on to the next step. If the sausage is still hot, then it will cook the egg when added to it after this step.

5. To the sausage mixture, add the eggs, baking powder, cheese, and coconut flour.

6. Combine well to incorporate. After the ingredients are thoroughly mixed, allow them to cool down for ten minutes. The flour will continue absorbing the mixture.

7. On an adequately greased baking sheet, place the cheese bites and sausage-egg mixture. Keep them arranged in rows. Bake them for twenty minutes.

Notes: *You must chill the dough before adding in the egg mixture, as avoiding this step would lead to flat bites.*

Sheet Pan Chicken Fajitas

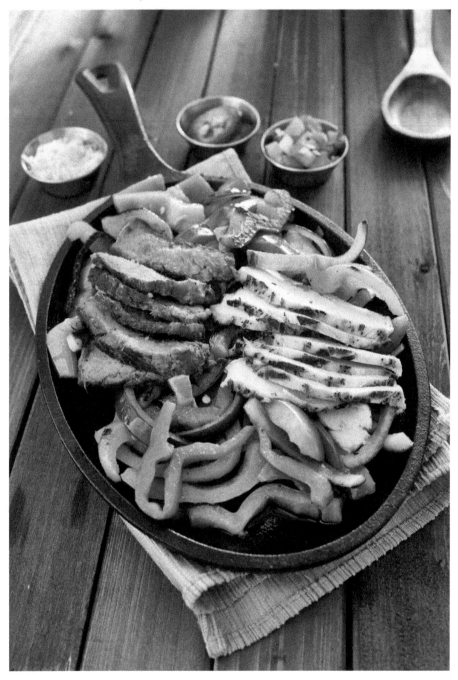

Total Prep & Cooking Time: 30 minutes

Yields: Six servings

Nutrition Facts: Calories: 357 | Carbs: 32.5g | Protein: 30.1g | Fat: 12.1g | Fiber: 6g

Ingredients:

- A quarter cup of taco seasoning
- One lime juiced
- One thinly sliced red onion
- One thinly chopped bell pepper (yellow)
- Small-sized tortillas (made of flour and warmed), optional
- Avocado
- Hot sauce
- Cilantro
- One tablespoon of olive oil
- Two pounds of chicken breasts (skinless and boneless, sliced into thin pieces)
- One bell pepper, red (chopped thinly)
- One green bell pepper (thinly chopped)

Method:

1. Take a large-sized bowl and add the lime juice, taco seasoning, and olive oil. Whisk this mixture together to form a marinade.

2. Then add the red onion, bell peppers (red, green, and yellow) and the chicken pieces to the marinade. Combine them thoroughly with a spoon. You should whisk the ingredients properly so that everything is mixed well. You can bake it at the very moment but, you can marinate for one hour before starting with the baking process to get a better taste.

3. Set the oven at a temperature of 375 degrees Fahrenheit for preheating.

4. Now take a sheet pan (preferably a rimmed one). On the sheet pan, arrange veggies and baked chicken. Bake for another twenty minutes until you cook the chicken thoroughly. If you like to have it overcooked, then broil for another three minutes.

5. After it is done, transfer them to serving plates. Garnish with hot sauce, tortillas (warmed), sour cream, avocado, and top with fresh cilantro.

6. Have it warm and enjoy it.

Chicken Shawarma Kebab

Total Prep & Cooking Time: 1 hour 10 minutes

Yields: Six servings

Nutrition Facts: Calories: 475 | Carbs: 48g | Protein: 41.6g | Fat: 13.2g | Fiber: 4.2g

Ingredients:

- Three pounds of chicken thigh (skinless and boneless)
- Two teaspoons each of
  - Cumin
  - Turmeric
  - Salt
  - Cardamom
  - Cinnamon
- One cup of yogurt (plain Greek)
- Parsley, fresh (optional)

For preparing the Tahini sauce,

- One cup of tahini (simple truth)
- Four cloves of garlic, diced
- One teaspoon of salt
- Half a cup of lemon juice
- One cup of water

Method:

1. Cut the chicken thigh into pieces of one inch each.

2. Take a bowl and place the yogurt, cardamom, cumin, turmeric, salt, and cinnamon. Add the sliced chicken pieces and then toss them properly. Combine with the help of spoon so that they can incorporate well. Cover the bowl with a lid or wrap the mouth with a paper completely and place it inside the refrigerator. Allow it to stay there for one hour.

3. Skewer the meat tightly with the help of metal skewers or soaked bamboo.

4. Keep the grill preheated to moderate heat. Place the marinated skewers on the rack and then cook the chicken thoroughly. Flip the pieces very often to ensure even cooking.

5. Take a small bowl and combine the ingredients for preparing the tahini sauce as listed above. Continue to stir the ingredients for one minute, even if they keep separating. After some time, they won't.

6. Serve the chicken with the tahini sauce and with cucumber and tomato.

One-Pan Cabbage Casserole

Total Prep & Cooking Time: 20 minutes

Yields: Six servings

Nutrition Facts: Calories: 240 | Carbs: 9g | Protein: 18.9g | Fat: 14.4g | Fiber: 1.6g

Ingredients:

- One lb. of turkey or beef (ground, drained, and browned)
- Half the head of cabbage (diced to form medium-sized chunks), approximately three cups
- Eighteen oz. of tomato sauce
- Pepper
- Salt
- One tsp. each of
  - Garlic powder
  - Chili powder
- One cup of cheese, shredded
- One small-sized onion, minced
- One can of green chilies with tomatoes

Method:

1. Turn the flame to moderate heat, place a skillet over it, and pour some oil. Add the turkey or beef to the oil and cook to make them brown. Drain off the extra grease.

2. Then add onion and stir for three to five minutes.

3. Add the tomatoes, tomato sauce, cabbage, green chilies, and the spices. Stir them well.

4. Cover the skillet and reduce the heat. Simmer for eighteen minutes and keep stirring occasionally.

5. Top the preparation with cheese and serve.

Chapter 4: One-Week Meal Plan

Here is a one-week meal plan to help you plan your days.

Monday

Breakfast – Tropical Smoothie Bowl

Lunch – Strawberry Salad

Dinner – Sheet Pan Chicken Fajitas

Snacks – Peanut Butter Balls

Tuesday

Breakfast – Banana Pancakes

Lunch – Cajun Shrimp Caesar Salad

Dinner – Zucchini Noodles and Turkey Meatballs

Snacks – Low Carb Green Smoothie

Wednesday

Breakfast – Breakfast Yogurt Parfait

Lunch – BLT Chicken Salad

Dinner – Sheet Pan Chicken Fajitas

Snacks – Peanut Butter Balls

Thursday

Breakfast – Tropical Smoothie Bowl

Lunch – Strawberry Salad

Dinner – Rosemary-Lemon Chicken

Snacks – Low Carb Green Smoothie

Friday

Breakfast – Smoked Salmon and Avocado Omelet

Lunch – BLT Chicken Salad

Dinner – Cucumber Salmon Panzanella

Snacks – Low Carb Cheesecake

Saturday

Breakfast – Breakfast Yogurt Parfait

Lunch – Mushroom and Asparagus Frittata

Dinner – Zucchini Noodles and Turkey Meatballs

Snacks – Peanut Butter Balls

Sunday

Breakfast – Tropical Smoothie Bowl

Lunch – One-Pan Cabbage Casserole

Dinner – Black Beans and Chicken Chili

Snacks – Egg, Sausage, and Cheese Bites

Resources

Alice A Gibson, A. S. (2017). Strategies to Improve Adherence to Dietary Weight Loss Interventions in Research and Real-World Settings. *Behavioral Sciences, 7*(4), 44.

Kathrin Pallauf, K. G. (2013). Nutrition and Healthy Ageing: Calorie Restriction or Polyphenol-Rich "MediterrAsian" Diet? *Oxidative Medicine and Cellular Longevity*, 1-14.

Manfred J. Müller, J. E.-W. (2016). Changes in Energy Expenditure with Weight Gain and Weight Loss in Humans. *Current Obesity Reports, 5*(4), 413-423.

Nawal Alajmi, K. D.-O. (2016). Appetite and Energy Intake Responses to Acute Energy Deficits in Females versus Males. *Medicine & Science in Sports & Exercise, 48*(3), 412-420.

Nawal Alajmi, K. D.-O. (2016). Appetite and Energy Intake Responses to Acute Energy Deficits in Females versus Males. *Medicine & Science in Sports & Exercise, 48*(3), 412-420.

Olivia M. Farr, M. C. (2015). New research developments and insights from Metabolism. *Metabolism, 64*(3), 354-367.

Pin-Hao Andy Chen, R. S. (2016). Structural integrity between executive control and reward regions of the brain predicts body fat percentage in chronic dieters. *Cognitive Neuroscience, 8*(3), 162-166.

Premawardhana, L. D. (2006). Management of thyroid disorders. *Postgraduate Medical Journal, 82*(971), 552-558.

Robert V. Considine, M. K. (1996). Serum Immunoreactive-Leptin Concentrations in Normal-Weight and Obese Humans. *New England Journal of Medicine, 334*(5), 292-295.

Sergiy Libert, L. G. (2013). Metabolic and Neuropsychiatric Effects of Calorie Restriction and Sirtuins. *Annual Review of Physiology, 75*(1), 669-684.

PART II

Are you worried that your hormones are not at their optimal levels? Here is a diet that will solve your problems.

Chapter 1: Health Benefits of the Hormone Diet

When it comes to getting healthy through weight loss, there's never any shortage of fitness crazes and diets that claim to have the secret to easy and sustainable weight loss. One of the latest diet plans that have come into the spotlight is the hormone diet, which claims that people often struggle to lose weight because of their hormones.

A hormone diet is a 3-step process that spans over six weeks and is designed to synchronize your hormones and promote a healthy body through detoxification, nutritional supplements, exercise, and diet. The diet controls what you eat and informs you about the correct time to eat to ensure maximum benefits to your hormones. Many books have been written on this topic with supporters of the diet assuring people that they can lose weight quickly and significantly through diet and exercise and reset or manipulate their hormones. Although the diet has a few variations, the central idea around each is that correcting the body's perceived hormonal imbalances is the key to losing weight.

The most important benefit of a hormone diet is that it takes a solid stance on improving overall health through weight loss and promoting regular exercise as well as natural, nutritious foods. Apart from that, it also focuses on adequate sleep, stress management, emotional health, and other healthy lifestyle habits that are all essential components that people should follow, whether it's a part of a diet or not. Including a water diet, it aims towards losing about twelve pounds in the 1st phase and 2 pounds a week after that.

Hormones have an essential role in the body's everyday processes, like helping bones grow, digesting food, etc. They act as "chemical messengers," instructing the cells to perform specific actions and are transported around the body through the bloodstream.

One of the very important food items to be included in the hormone diet is salmon. Salmon is rich in omega-3 fatty acids, Docosahexaenoic acid, and Eicosapentaenoic acid (EPA). It is rich in selenium too. These help to lower your blood pressure and also reduce the level of unhealthy cholesterol in the blood. These make you less prone to heart diseases. Salmon is a rich source of healthy fat. If consumed in sufficient amounts, it provides you energy and helps you get rid of unwanted body fat. Salmon is well-known for giving fantastic weight loss results as it has less saturated fat, unlike other protein sources. Salmon is packed with vitamins like vitamin-k, E, D, and A. These are extremely helpful for your eyes, bone joints, etc. These vitamins are also good for your brain, regulation of metabolic balance, and repairing your muscles. Salmon's vitamins and omega-3 fatty acids are amazing for sharpening your mind. It also improves your memory retention power. If you consume salmon, you are less likely to develop dementia or mental dis-functions. Salmon has anti-inflammatory properties and is low in omega-6 fatty acid content (which is pro-inflammatory in nature and is present in a huge amount in the modern diet). It promotes healthy skin and gives you radiant and glowing skin. It is good for the winter because it helps you to stay warm. It also provides lubrication to your joints because of the abundant presence of essential minerals and fatty acids in it. Apart from this, some other things to include in your diet are arugula, kale, ginger, avocado, carrots, and so on.

There are almost sixteen hormones that can influence weight. For example, the hormone leptin produced by your fat cells is considered a "satiety hormone," which makes you feel full by reducing your appetite. As a signaling hormone, it communicates with the part of your brain (hypothalamus) that controls food intake and appetite. Leptin informs the brain when there is enough fat in storage, and extra fat is not required. This helps prevent overeating. Individuals who are obese or overweight generally have very high levels of leptin in their blood. Research shows that the level of leptin in obese individuals was almost four times higher than that in individuals with normal weight.

Studies have found that fat hormones like leptin and adiponectin can promote long-term weight loss by reducing appetite and increasing metabolism. It is believed that both these fat hormones follow the same pathway in the brain to manage blood sugar (glucose) and body weight (Robert V. Considine, 1996).

Simply put, the hormone diet works by helping to create a calorie deficit through better nutritional habits and exercise, which ultimately results in weight loss. It's also essential to consult a doctor before following this detox diet or consuming any dietary supplements.

Chapter 2: Hormone-Rebalancing Smoothies

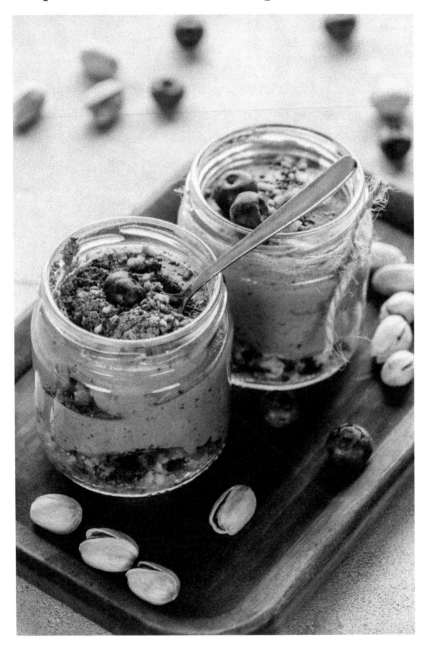

Estrogen Detox Smoothie

Total Prep & Cooking Time: 5 minutes

Yields: One glass

Nutrition Facts: Calories: 312 | Carbs: 47.9g | Protein: 18.6g | Fat: 8.5g | Fiber: 3g

Ingredients:

- Half a cup of hemp seeds
- Two kiwis (medium-sized)
- A quarter each of
  o   Avocado (medium-sized)
  o   Cucumber (medium-sized)
- Half a unit each of
  o   Lemon (squeezed freshly)
  o   Green apple
- One celery (medium-sized)
- A quarter cup of cilantro
- Two tbsps. of chis seeds
- Two cups of water (filtered)
- One tsp. of cacao nibs
- One tbsp. of coconut oil

Method:

1. Blend the ingredients all together to form a smoothie at high speed. The thickness can be adjusted according to your preference by adding more water to the mixture.

2. Serve and enjoy.

Dopamine Delight Smoothie

Total Prep Time: 10 minutes

Yields: One serving

Nutrition Facts: Calories: 383 | Carbs: 31g | Protein: 24g | Fat: 18.g | Fiber: 3g

Ingredients:

- Half a teaspoon of cinnamon (ground)
- Half a cup of peeled banana (the bananas must be frozen)
- One organic espresso, double shot (measuring half a cup)
- One tablespoon of chia seeds
- A three-fourth cup of soy milk (plain or vanilla-flavored)
- Protein powder, a serving (from the whey with the flavor of vanilla)

Method:

1. Fill in the bowl of your blender with all the ingredients (from the section of ingredients) except the whey protein powder and then proceed by switching to a high-speed blending option. Make sure it acquires a smooth consistency and then pour it out.

2. Now you may add the protein powder and give it another shot of blend until the whole things get incorporated, a bit of the goat cheese (already crumbled).

Breakfast Smoothie Bowl

Total Prep Time: 10 minutes

Yields: 2 servings

Nutrition Facts: Calories: 290 | Carbs: 53g | Protein: 6g | Fat: 8g | Fiber: 9g

Ingredients:

- One cup of thoroughly rinsed blueberries (fresh and ripe)
- A sundry of nuts and fruits for garnishing, which includes – strawberries, bananas (thinly sliced), peanuts (Spanish), kiwi (chopped), segments of tangerine, and raspberries.
- One cup of Greek yogurt

For the preparation of honey flax granola,

- Two tablespoons each of
  - o Flaxseeds
  - o Vegetable oil
- Oats (old-fashioned), approximately a cup
- One tablespoon of honey

Method:

1. Set your oven at a temperature of 350 degrees F.

2. Preparation of the smoothie: collect the diverse types of berries, wash them thoroughly, and then put them in the blender and turn it on. Make an even mixture out of it. Add some amount of the yogurt and blend it again to form a smooth texture.

3. For preparing the granola: Take a small-sized bowl and then drizzle a few drops oil in it. Then add the oats, flax, and honey to the oil, one by one, and mix it well. You are required to toss the bowl thoroughly to get the mixture well-coated with the poured oil. After you are done, place the oats mixture in a baking sheet evenly. Bake it for about twenty minutes. This mark will be enough to give the oats a beautiful tinge of golden brown. Allow it to cool.

4. Now you will require a shallow bowl to spoon in some yogurt, and this will be the first layer. Form a second layer with the various fruits and nuts and finally for the third layer, top with the granola.

5. Enjoy.

Notes:

- *Using frozen nuts and fruits in a warm-weather will get much to your relief.*

- *For a vegan smoothie bowl, sub the yogurt with coconut or almond yogurt.*

- *Give the pan a few strokes while baking the oats.*

Blueberry Detox Smoothie

Total Prep Time: Ten minutes

Yields: One serving

Nutrition Facts: Calories: 326 | Carbs: 65g | Protein: 4g | Fat: 8g | Fiber: 9g

Ingredients:

- One cup of wild blueberries (frozen)
- One banana (sliced into several pieces) frozen
- Orange juice (approximately half a cup)
- Cilantro leaves, fresh (approximately a measuring a small handful size)
- A quarter of an entire avocado
- A quarter cup of water

Method:

1. Add cilantro, avocado, water, blueberries, banana, and orange juice in the blender and then process.

2. Make the ingredients integrated so well that they become smooth in their consistency.

Notes: *It is recommended that you add the potent herb, cilantro, or parsley in a small amount when consuming this smoothie for the first time, as it might trigger a mild headache. If you do not get a headache, you may add a bit more of the cilantro leaves.*

Maca Mango Smoothie

Total Prep & Cooking Time: 2 minutes

Yields: 2 servings

Nutrition Facts: Calories: 53 | Carbs: 13g | Protein: 1g | Fat: 3g | Fiber: 1.5g

Ingredients:

- One and a half cups each of
  - Fresh mango
  - Frozen mango
- One tablespoon each of
  - Ground flaxseed
  - Nut butter
- One teaspoon of ground turmeric
- Two teaspoons of maca root powder
- Three-quarter cups of nut milk
- One frozen banana

Method:

1. Blend all the ingredients together to get a smooth mixture.

2. Adjust consistency by adding nut milk.

3. Once done, divide into two glasses and enjoy!

Pituitary Relief Smoothie

Total Prep & Cooking Time: 5 minutes

Yields: 2 servings

Nutrition Facts: Calories: 174 | Carbs: 18.3g | Protein: 9.7g | Fat: 8.3g | Fiber: 14.4g

Ingredients:

- One teaspoon of coconut oil
- One fresh or frozen ripe banana
- One tablespoon of raw sesame seeds
- Two teaspoons each of
  - Chia seeds
  - Raw Maca powder
  - Raw Spirulina
- Two cups of water
- Two tablespoons of hulled hemp seeds

Method:

1. You have to use a blender to process this smoothie. Add the hulled hemp seeds, sesame seeds, and water in the blender and process them. Do it at high speed, and it will only require a minute. This will give you raw-milk like texture.

2. Then, add the following ingredients into it – coconut oil, banana, chia seeds, Maca, and Spirulina, and process the ingredients once again but this time on medium speed for another minute or so. Everything will become well incorporated.

3. You have to drink this smoothie on an empty stomach.

Notes: *In order to make the smoothie rich in antioxidants, you can add some fresh fruits like blueberries, kiwi, and raspberries.*

Chapter 2: Easy Breakfast Recipes

Scrambled Eggs With Feta and Tomatoes

Total Prep & Cooking Time: 10 minutes

Yields: One Plate

Nutrition Facts: Calories: 421 | Carbs: 8.6g | Protein: 20.3g | Fat: 35.1g | Fiber: 1.6g

Ingredients:

- One tbsp. each of
  - Olive oil (extra virgin)
  - Freshly chopped parsley, basil, dill or chives
- Half a cup of cherry tomatoes (each tomato sliced into half)
- Two ounces of crumbled feta cheese (approximately a quarter cup)
- Two eggs are beaten
- Two tbsp. of onion (diced)
- To taste:
  - Black pepper
  - Kosher salt

Method:

1. Keep the beaten eggs in a small-sized bowl and then season it with a pinch of pepper and salt. Set the bowl aside.

2. Use a nonstick skillet to proceed with the cooking. Pour two tbsp. of olive oil. Then add the diced onions. Stir over moderate heat and cook until softened. Make sure that the onions do not look brown. This process should get done by a minute.

3. Add half a cup of tomatoes to skillet and then continue to mix for about two minutes.

4. Now you may add the eggs. Using a spatula, gather the beaten eggs to the center by moving spatula all over the skillet.

5. The eggs will take an additional minute to get cooked. So after that mark, add the parsley or other herbs (if preferred) and feta cheese. Keep the eggs underdone as they will get cooked completely after they are served in the plate itself (from the residual heat). Therefore, cook the entire thing in the skillet for 30 seconds only.

6. Take a serving plate and transfer the eggs to it. Top with some sprinkled parsley and feta cheese, drizzled with some oil, and seasoned with some pepper and salt. These additions are optional and may vary as per your desire.

Smashed Avo and Quinoa

Total Prep & Cooking Time: 15 minutes

Yields: Six bowls

Nutrition Facts: Calories: 492 | Carbs: 67g | Protein: 15g | Fat: 20g | Fiber: 13g

Ingredients:

- One avocado skinned, cut into half, and then pitted
- A handful of cilantro or coriander
- Half a lemon (juiced)
- A quarter red onion (diced finely)
- One-eighth teaspoon of cayenne pepper
- To taste: Sea salt

For the Greens,

- One handful of kale
- One handful of soft herbs (basil, parsley or mint)
- One handful of chard or spinach
- For frying: butter or coconut oil

Serve with,

- One cup of quinoa (cooked)

Method:

1. You will require a frying pan to get this done. To it, add the coconut oil or butter (whichever you prefer) and add the greens. Toss them carefully and then sauté over moderate heat. Stop when they become soft.

2. Mix the onion, cayenne, avocado, cilantro, salt, lemon, and pepper to a bowl and mix them completely. The pepper and salt must be added according to the taste.

3. Add cooked quinoa to the tossed greens and heat altogether over low heat.

4. Take a serving plate and place the quinoa mixture and greens to it. Crown the whole thing with smashed avocado and then serve.

Hormone Balancing Granola

Total Prep & Cooking Time: 35 minutes

Yields: 8 servings

Nutrition Facts: Calories: 360 | Carbs: 19.8g | Protein: 5.1g | Fat: 28.8g | Fiber: 5.8g

Ingredients:

- One-third cup each of
  - Flaxseed meal
  - Pumpkin seeds
  - Seedless raisins
- Two teaspoons of cinnamon
- One teaspoon of vanilla extract
- Four tablespoons of maple syrup
- Five tablespoons of melted coconut oil
- A quarter cup of unsweetened coconut flakes
- Two-thirds cup each of
  - Chopped pecans
  - Chopped brazil nuts
- Two tablespoons of ground chia seeds

Method:

1. Set the temperature of the oven to 180 degrees F and preheat.

2. In a food processor, chop the pecans and the Brazil nuts. Then, mix these chopped nuts with coconut flakes, seeds, and other nuts present in the list of ingredients.

3. Add maple syrup, coconut oil, cinnamon, and vanilla extract in a separate bowl and combine well.

4. Now, take the wet ingredients and pour them into the dry ingredients. Mix thoroughly so that everything has become coated properly.

5. Place the prepared mixture in the oven for half an hour and cook.

6. Once done, cut into pieces and serve.

Chapter 3: Healthy Lunch Recipes

Easy Shakshuka

Total Prep & Cooking Time: 30 minutes

Yields: Six servings

Nutrition Facts: Calories: 154 | Carbs: 4.1g | Protein: 9g | Fat: 7.8g | Fiber: 0g

Ingredients:

- Olive oil (extra virgin)
- Two chopped green peppers
- One teaspoon each of
  - Paprika (sweet)
  - Coriander (ground)
- A pinch of red pepper (flakes)
- Half a cup of tomato sauce
- A quarter cup each of
  - Mint leaves (freshly chopped)
  - Parsley leaves (chopped freshly)
- One yellow onion, large-sized (chopped)
- Two cloves of garlic, chopped
- Half a teaspoon of cumin (ground)
- Six cups of chopped tomatoes (Vine-ripe)
- Six large-sized eggs

- To taste: Pepper and salt

Method:

1. You will require a large-sized skillet (made of cast iron). Pour three tablespoons of oil and heat it. After bringing the oil to boil, add the peppers, spices, onions, garlic, pepper, and salt. Stir time to time to cook the veggies for five minutes until they become softened.

2. After the vegetables become soft, add the chopped tomatoes and then tomato sauce. Cover the skillet and simmer for an additional fifteen minutes.

3. Now, you may remove the lid from the pan and then cook a touch more to thicken the consistency. At this point, you may adjust the taste.

4. Make six cavities within the tomato mixture and crack one egg each inside the cavities.

5. Cover the skillet after reducing the heat and allow it to cook so that the eggs settle into the cavities.

6. Keep track of the time and accordingly uncover the skillet and then add mint and parsley. Season with more black and red pepper according to your desire. Serve them warm with the sort of bread you wish.

Ginger Chicken

Total Prep & Cooking Time: 50 minutes

Yields: Six Servings

Nutrition Facts: Calories: 310 | Carbs: 6g | Protein: 37g | Fat: 16g | Fiber: 1g

Ingredients:

- A one-kilogram pack of chicken thighs (skinless and boneless)
- Four cloves of garlic (chopped finely)
- A fifteen-gram pack of coriander (fresh and chopped)
- Two tablespoons of sunflower oil
- One teaspoon each of
  - Turmeric (ground)
  - Chili powder (mild)
- A four hundred milliliter can of coconut milk (reduced-fat)
- One cube of chicken stock
- One ginger properly peeled and chopped finely (it should be of the size of a thumb)
- One lime, juiced
- Two medium-sized onions
- One red chili, sliced and the seeds removed (fresh)

Method:

1. Make the chicken thighs into three large chunks and marinate them with chili powder, garlic, coriander (half of the entire amount), ginger, oil (one tbsp.), and lime juice. Cover the bowl after stirring them well and then store it in the fridge until oven-ready.

2. Marinade the chicken and keep overnight for better flavor.

3. Chop the onions finely (it is going to be the simplest for preparing the curry) before dropping them into the food processor. Pour oil into the frying pan (large-sized) and heat it. Then add chopped onions and stir them thoroughly for eight minutes until the pieces become soft. Then pour the turmeric powder and stir for an additional minute.

4. Now add the chicken mixture and cook on high heat until you notice a change in its color. Pour the chicken stock, chili, and coconut milk and after covering the pan simmer for another twenty minutes. Sprinkle the left-over coriander leaves and then serve hot.

5. Enjoy.

Carrot and Miso Soup

Total Prep & Cooking Time: 1 hour

Yields: Four bowls of soup

Nutrition Facts: Calories: 76 | Carbs: 8.76g | Protein: 4.83g | Fat: 2.44g | Fiber: 1.5g

Ingredients:

- Two tbsps. of oil
- Garlic, minced (four cloves)
- One inch of garlic (grated)
- Three tbsps. of miso paste (white)
- One diced onion
- One pound of carrot (sliced thinly)
- Four cups of vegetable stock
- To taste: Pepper and Salt

For garnishing,

- Two scallions (sliced thinly)
- Chili pepper (seven spices)
- One nori roasted (make thin slivers)
- Sesame oil

Method:

1. Using a soup pot will be convenient to proceed with. Pour oil in a pot and then heat over a high flame. Now you may put garlic, carrot, and onion and sauté them thoroughly. Cook for about ten minutes so that the onions turn translucent.

2. Then add the ginger and vegetable stock. Mix them well and cook all together. Put the flame to simmer. Cover the pot while cooking to make the carrot tender. This will take another thirty minutes.

3. Put off the flame and puree the soup with the help of an immersion blender.

4. Use a small-sized bowl to whisk together a spoonful of the soup and the white miso paste. Stir until the paste dissolve and pour the mixture back to the pot.

5. Add pepper and salt if required.

6. Divide the soup among four bowls and enrich its feel by adding scallions, sesame oil, seven spices, and nori.

Arugula Salad

Total Prep & Cooking Time: 1 hour 10 minutes

Yields: Two bowls of salad

Nutrition Facts: Calories: 336.8 | Carbs: 30.6g | Protein: 7.7g | Fat: 22.2g | Fiber: 7.3g

Ingredients:

For the salad,

- Two medium-sized beets (boiled or roasted for about an hour), skinned and sliced into pieces that can easily be bitten
- Four tablespoons of goat cheese
- Approximately 2.5 oz. of baby arugula (fresh)
- A quarter cup of walnuts (chopped roughly before toasting)

For the dressing,

- Three tablespoons of olive oil (extra virgin)
- A quarter tsp. each of
    o   Mustard powder (dried)
    o   Pepper
- Half a tsp. each of
    o   Salt
    o   Sugar

- One and a half tablespoons of lemon juice

Method:

1. For preparing the vinaigrette, place all the ingredients (listed in the dressing ingredients section) in a jar and then shake them to emulsify. At this stage, before starting with the process of emulsification, you may add or remove the ingredients as per your liking.

2. Get the salad assembled (again depending upon the taste you want to give it), add a fistful of arugula leaves, place some chopped beets (after they have been cooked), and finally the toasted walnuts (already chopped).

3. Drizzle vinaigrette over the salad and enjoy.

Notes:

- *Coat the beets with oil (olive), roll them up in an aluminum foil, and then roast the beets at a temperature of 400 degrees F.*

- *And for boiling the beets, immerse them in water after transferring to a pot and simmer them for 45 minutes.*

Kale Soup

Total Prep & Cooking Time: 55 minutes

Yields: 8 servings

Nutrition Facts: Calories: 277.3 | Carbs: 50.9g | Protein: 9.6g | Fat: 4.5g | Fiber: 10.3g

Ingredients:

- Two tbsps. of dried parsley
- One tbsp. of Italian seasoning
- Salt and pepper
- Thirty oz. of drained cannellini beans
- Six peeled and cubed white potatoes
- Fifteen ounces of diced tomatoes
- Six vegetable Bouillon cubes
- Eight cups of water
- One bunch of kale (with chopped leaves and stems removed)
- Two tbsps. of chopped garlic
- One chopped yellow onion
- Two tbsps. of olive oil

Method:

1. At first, take a large soup pot, add in some olive oil, and heat it.

2. Add garlic and onion. Cook them until soft.

3. Then stir in the kale and cook for about two minutes, until wilted.

4. Pour the water and add the beans, potatoes, tomatoes, vegetable bouillon, parsley, and the Italian seasoning.

5. On medium heat, simmer the soup for about twenty-five minutes, until the potatoes are cooked through.

6. Finally, do the seasoning with salt and pepper according to your taste.

Roasted Sardines

Total Prep & Cooking Time: 25 minutes

Yields: 4 servings

Nutrition Facts: Calories: 418 | Carbs: 2.6g | Protein: 41g | Fat: 27.2g | Fiber: 0.8g

Ingredients:

- 3.5 oz. of cherry tomatoes (cut them in halves)
- One medium-sized red onion (chopped finely)
- Two tablespoons each of
  - Chopped parsley
  - Extra-virgin olive oil
- One clove of garlic (halved)
- Eight units of fresh sardines (gutted and cleaned, heads should be cleaned)
- A quarter teaspoon of chili flakes
- One teaspoon of toasted cumin seeds
- Half a lemon (zested and juiced)

Method:

1. Set the temperature of the oven to 180 degrees C and preheat. Take a roasting tray and grease it lightly.

2.   Take a bowl and add the tomatoes and onions in it. Add the lemon juice too and toss the veggies in the lemon juice. Now, add the zest, olive oil, chili, cumin, garlic, and parsley and toss everything once again.

3.   Use pepper and salt to season the mixture. The cavity of the sardines has to be filled. Use some of the tomato and onion mixture for this purpose. Once done, place the sardines on the prepared roasting tray. Take the remaining mixture and scatter it over the sardines.

4.   Roast the sardines for about 10-15 minutes, and by the end of this, they should be cooked thoroughly.

5.   Serve and enjoy!

Chapter 4: Tasty Dinner Recipes

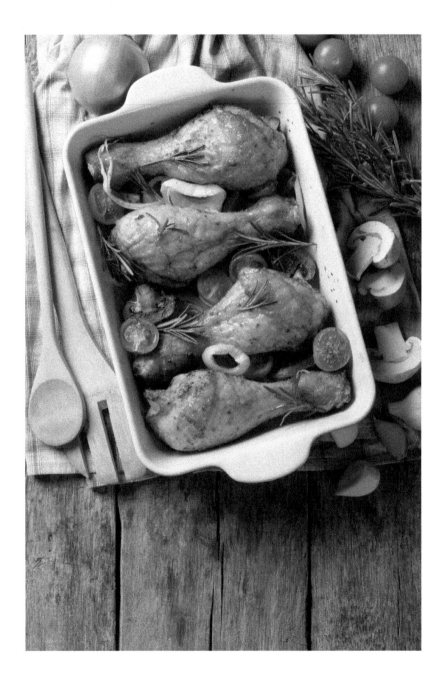

Rosemary Chicken

Total Prep & Cooking Time: 50 minutes

Yields: 4 servings

Nutrition Facts: Calories: 232 | Carbs: 3.9g | Protein: 26.7g | Fat: 11.6g | Fiber: 0.3g

Ingredients:

- Four chicken breast halves (skinless and boneless)
- One-eighth tsp. kosher salt
- One-fourth tsp. ground black pepper
- One and a half tbsps. of lemon juice
- One and a half tbsps. of Dijon mustard
- Two tbsps. of freshly minced rosemary
- Three tbsps. of olive oil
- Eight minced garlic cloves

Method:

1. At first, preheat a grill to medium-high heat. The grate needs to be lightly oiled.

2. Take a bowl and add lemon juice, mustard, rosemary, olive oil, garlic, salt, and ground black pepper. Whisk them together.

3. Take a resealable plastic bag and place the chicken breasts in it. Over the chicken, pour the garlic mixture (reserve one-eighth cup of it).

4. Seal the bag and start massaging the marinade gently into the chicken. Allow it to stand for about thirty minutes at room temperature.

5. Then on the preheated grill, place the chicken and cook for about four minutes.

6. Flip the chicken and baste it with the marinade reserved and then cook for about five minutes, until thoroughly cooked.

Finally, cover it with a foil and allow it to rest for about 2 minutes before you serve them.

Corned Beef and Cabbage
Total Prep & Cooking Time: 2 hours 35 minutes

Yields: 5 servings

Nutrition Facts: Calories: 868.8 | Carbs: 75.8g | Protein: 50.2g | Fat: 41.5g | Fiber: 14g

Ingredients:

- One big cabbage head (cut it into small wedges)
- Five peeled carrots (chopped into three-inch pieces)
- Ten red potatoes (small)
- Three pounds of corned beef brisket (along with the packet of spice)

Method:

1. At first, in a Dutch oven or a large pot, place the corned beef, and cover it with water. Then add in the spices from the packet of spices that came along with the beef. Cover the pot, bring it to a boil, and finally reduce it to a simmer. Allow it to simmer for about 2 hours and 30 minutes or until tender.

2. Add carrots and whole potatoes, and cook them until the vegetables are tender. Add the cabbage wedges and cook for another fifteen minutes. Then finally remove the meat and allow it to rest for fifteen minutes.

3. Take a bowl, place the vegetables in it, and cover it. Add broth (which is reserved in the pot) as much as you want. Then finally cut the meat against the grain.

Roasted Parsnips and Carrots

Total Prep & Cooking Time: 1 hour

Yields: 4 servings

Nutrition Facts: Calories: 112 | Carbs: 27g | Protein: 2g | Fat: 1g | Fiber: 7g

Ingredients:

- Two tbsps. of freshly minced parsley or dill
- One and a half tsp. of freshly ground black pepper
- One tbsp. kosher salt
- Three tbsps. of olive oil
- One pound of unpeeled carrots
- Two pounds of peeled parsnips

Method:

1. At first, preheat your oven to 425 degrees.

2. If the carrots and parsnips are thick, then cut them into halves lengthwise.

3. Then, slice each of them diagonally into one inch thick slices. Don't cut them too small because the vegetables will anyway shrink while you cook them.

4. Take a sheet pan, and place the cut vegetables on it.

5. Then add some olive oil, pepper, salt, and toss them nicely.

6. Roast them for about twenty to forty minutes (the roasting time depends on the size of the vegetables), accompanied by occasional tossing. Continue to roast until the carrots and parsnips become tender.

7. Finally, sprinkle some dill and serve.

Herbed Salmon

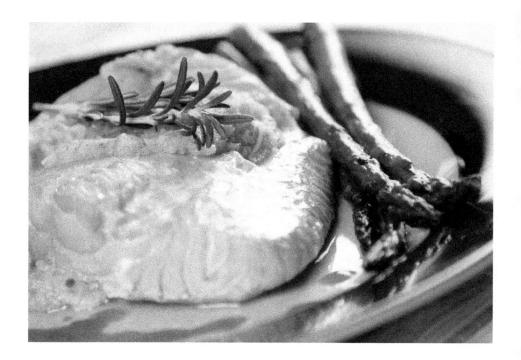

Total Prep & Cooking Time: 30 minutes

Yields: 4 servings

Nutrition Facts: Calories: 301 | Carbs: 1g | Protein: 29g | Fat: 19g | Fiber: 0g

Ingredients:

- Half a tsp. of dried thyme or two tsps. of freshly minced thyme
- Half a tsp. of pepper

- Three-fourth tsp. of salt
- One tbsp. of olive oil
- One tbsp. freshly minced rosemary or one tsp. of crushed dried rosemary.
- Four minced cloves of garlic
- Four (six ounces) fillets of salmon

Method:

1. At first, preheat your oven to 425 degrees.

2. Take a 15 by 10 by 1 inch baking pan and grease it.

3. Place the salmon on it while keeping the skin side down.

4. Combine the garlic cloves, rosemary, thyme, salt, and pepper. Spread it evenly over the salmon fillets.

5. Roast them for about fifteen to eighteen minutes until they reach your desired doneness.

Chipotle Cauliflower Tacos

Total Prep & Cooking Time: 30 minutes

Yields: 8 servings

Nutrition Facts: Calories: 440 | Carbs: 51.6g | Protein: 10.1g | Fat: 24g | Fiber: 9g

Ingredients:

For the tacos,

- Four tablespoons of avocado oil
- One head of cauliflower (large-sized, chopped into bite-sized florets)
- One cup of cilantro (freshly chopped)
- One tablespoon each of
  - Fresh lime juice
  - Maple syrup or honey
- Two tsps. of chipotle adobo sauce
- Cracked black pepper
- One teaspoon of salt
- 4-8 units of garlic cloves (freshly minced)

For the Chipotle Aioli,

- A quarter cup of chipotle adobo sauce
- Half a cup each of
  - Sour cream
  - Clean mayo

One teaspoon of sea salt

Two cloves of garlic (minced)

For serving,

- Almond flour tortillas
- Guacamole
- Almond ricotta cheese
- Sliced tomatoes, radish, and cabbage

Method:

1. Set the temperature of the oven to 425 degrees F. Now, use parchment paper to line a pan. Take the bite-sized florets of the cauliflower and spread them evenly on the pan. Use 2-4 tbsps. of avocado oil, pepper, salt, and minced garlic and drizzle it on the pan.

2. Roast the cauliflower for half an hour at 425 degrees F and halfway through the process, flip the florets.

3. When you are roasting the cauliflower, take the rest of the ingredients of the cauliflower and mix them in a bowl. Once everything has been properly incorporated, set the mixture aside.

4. Now, take another bowl and in it, add the ingredients of the chipotle aioli. Mix them and set the bowl aside.

5. If you have any other taco fixings, get them ready.

6. Once the cauliflower is ready, toss the florets in the chipotle sauce.

7. Serve the cauliflower in tortillas along with fixings of your choice and the chipotle aioli.

-

PART III

The sirtfood diet is one of the latest diet patterns that has garnered quite the attention. The idea was brought to the market by two nutritionists Glen Matten and Aidan Goggins. The main idea of the diet revolves around sirtuins, which are basically a group of 7 proteins that are responsible for the functioning and regulation of lifespan, inflammation, and metabolism (Sergiy Libert, 2013).

Chapter 1: Health Benefits of the Diet

The benefits are vast. This includes loss in weight, better skin quality, gain in muscle mass in the areas that are very much required, increased metabolic rate, feeling of fullness without having to eat much (this is the power of the foods actually), suppressing the appetite, and leading a better and confident life. This specifically includes an increase in the memory, supporting the body to control blood sugar and blood cholesterol level in a much-advanced way, and wiping out the damage caused by the free radicals and thus preventing them from having adverse impacts on the cells that might lead to other diseases like cancer.

The consumption of these foods, along with the drinks, has a number of observational shreds of evidence that link the sirtfoods with the reducing hazards of several chronic diseases. This diet is notably suited as an anti-aging scheme. Sirtfoods have the ability to satiate the appetite in a natural way and increase the functioning of the muscle. These two points are enough to find a solution that can ultimately help us to achieve a healthy weight. In addition to this, the health-improving impact of these compounds is powerful in comparison to the drugs that are prescribed in order to prevent several chronic diseases like that of diabetes, heart problems, Alzheimer's, etc.

A pilot study was conducted on a total of 39 participants. At the end of the first week, the participants had an increase in muscle mass and also lost 7 pounds on average. Research has proven that in this initial week, the weight loss that is witnessed is mostly from water, glycogen, and muscle, and only one-third of it is from fat (Manfred J. Müller, 2016). The major sirtfoods include red wine, kale, soy, strawberries, matcha green tea, extra virgin olive oil, walnuts, buckwheat, capers, lovage, coffee, dark chocolate, Medjool dates, turmeric, red chicory, parsley, onions, arugula, and blueberries (Kathrin Pallauf, 2013).

Chapter 2: Sirtfood Juice Recipes

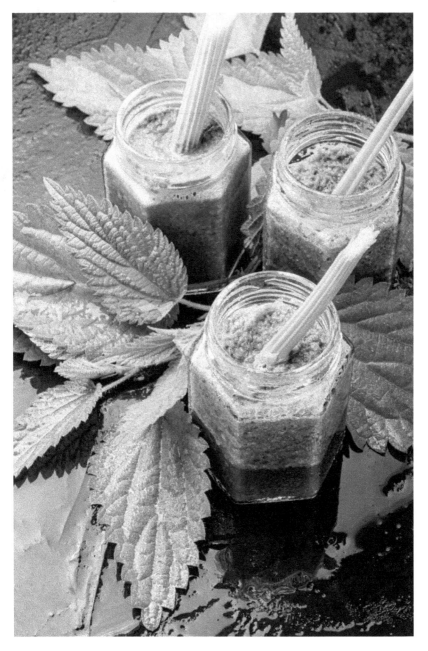

Green Juice

Total Prep & Cooking Time: Five minutes

Yields: 1 serving

Nutrition Facts: Calories: 182.3 | Carbs: 42.9g | Protein: 6g | Fat: 1.5g | Fiber: 12.7g

Ingredients:

- Half a green apple
- Two sticks of celery
- Five grams of parsley
- Thirty grams of rocket
- Seventy-five grams of kale
- Half a teaspoon of matcha green tea
- Juice of half a lemon
- One cm of ginger

Method:

1. Juice the kale, rocket, celery sticks, green apple, and parsley in a juicer.

2. Add the lemon juice into the green juice by squeezing it with your hand.

3. Take a glass and pour a little amount of the green juice into it. Add the matcha green tea and stir it in. Then, pour the remaining green juice into the glass and stir to combine everything properly.

4. You can choose to save it for later or drink it straight away.

Blueberry Kale Smoothie

Total Prep & Cooking Time: Five minutes

Yields: 1 serving

Nutrition Facts: Calories: 240 | Carbs: 37.9g | Protein: 17.2g | Fat: 3.6g | Fiber: 7g

Ingredients:

- Half a cup each of
    - o   Plain low-fat yogurt
    - o   Blueberries (frozen or fresh)
    - o   Kale, chopped
- Half a banana
- Half a teaspoon of cinnamon powder
- One tablespoon of flaxseed meal
- One scoop of protein powder
- Half a cup of water (optional)
- Two handfuls of ice (you can add more if you like)

Method:

1. Take a high-speed blender and add all the ingredients in it.

2. Blend everything together until you get a smooth puree.

3. Pour the blueberry kale smoothie in a glass and serve cold.

Tropical Kale Smoothie

Total Prep & Cooking Time: 10 minutes

Yields: 2 servings

Nutrition Facts: Calories: 187 | Carbs: 46.8g | Protein: 3.5g | Fat: 0.5g | Fiber: 4.7g

Ingredients:

- Half a cup to one cup of orange juice (about 120 ml to 240 ml)
- One banana, chopped (use frozen banana, is possible)
- Two cups of pineapple (about 330 grams), chopped (use frozen pineapple if possible)
- One and a half cups of kale (around 90 grams), chopped

Method:

1. Add the chopped bananas, pineapple, kale, and orange juice into a blender and blend everything together until you get a smooth puree.

2. You can add more orange juice if you need to attain a smoothie consistency. The amount of frozen fruit used directly affects the consistency of the smoothie.

3. Pour the smoothie equally into two glasses and serve cold.

Strawberry Oatmeal Smoothie

Total Prep & Cooking Time: 5 minutes

Yields: 2 servings

Nutrition Facts: Calories: 236.1 | Carbs: 44.9g | Protein: 7.6g | Fat: 3.7g | Fiber: 5.9g

Ingredients:

- Half a tsp. of vanilla extract
- Fourteen frozen strawberries
- One banana (cut into chunks)
- Half a cup of rolled oats
- One cup of soy milk
- One and a half tsps. of white sugar

Method:

1. Take a blender. Add the strawberries, banana, oats, and soy milk.
2. Then add sugar and vanilla extract.
3. Blend until the texture becomes smooth.
4. Then pour it into a glass and serve.

Chapter 3: Main Course Recipes for Sirtfood Diet

Green Juice Salad

Total Prep & Cooking Time: Ten minutes

Yields: 1 serving

Nutrition Facts: Calories: 199 | Carbs: 27g | Protein: 10g | Fat: 8.2g | Fiber: 9.2g

Ingredients:

- Six walnuts, halved
- Half of a green apple, sliced
- Two sticks of celery, sliced
- One tablespoon each of
  - Parsley
  - Olive oil
- One handful of rocket
- Two handfuls of kale, sliced
- One cm of ginger, grated
- Juice of half a lemon
- Salt and pepper to taste

Method:

1. To make the dressing, add the olive oil, ginger, lemon juice, salt, and pepper in a jam jar. Shake the jar to combine everything together.

2. Keep the sliced kale in a large bowl and add the dressing over it. Massage the dressing for about a minute to mix it with the kale properly.

3. Lastly, add the remaining ingredients (walnuts, sliced green apple, celery sticks, parsley, and rocket) into the bowl and combine everything thoroughly.

King Prawns and Buckwheat Noodles

Total Prep & Cooking Time: Twenty minutes

Yields: 4 servings

Nutrition Facts: Calories: 496 | Carbs: 53.2g | Protein: 22.2g | Fat: 17.6g | Fiber: 4.8g

Ingredients:

- 600 grams of king prawn
- 300 grams of soba or buckwheat noodles (using 100 percent buckwheat is recommended)
- One bird's eye chili, membranes, and seeds eliminated and finely chopped (and more according to taste)
- Three cloves of garlic, finely chopped or grated
- Three cm of ginger, grated
- 100 grams of green beans, chopped
- 100 grams of kale, roughly chopped
- Two celery sticks, sliced
- One red onion, thinly sliced
- Two tablespoons each of
  - Parsley, finely chopped (or lovage, if you have it)
  - Soy sauce or tamari (and extra for serving)
  - Extra virgin olive oil

Method:

1. Boil the buckwheat noodles for three to five minutes or until they are cooked according to your liking. Drain the water and then rinse the noodles in cold water. Drizzle some olive oil on the top and mix it with the noodles. Keep this mixture aside.

2. Prepare the remaining ingredients while the noodles are boiling.

3. Place a large frying pan or a wok over low heat and add a little olive oil into it. Then add the celery and red onions and fry them for about three minutes so that they get soft.

4. Then add the green beans and kale and increase the heat to medium-high. Fry them for about three minutes.

5. Decrease the heat again and then add the prawns, chili, ginger, and garlic into the pan. Fry for another two to three minutes so that the prawns get hot all the way through.

6. Lastly, add in the buckwheat noodles, soy sauce/tamari, and cook it for another minute so that the noodles get warm again.

7. Sprinkle some chopped parsley on the top as a garnish and serve hot.

Red Onion Dhal and Buckwheat

Total Prep & Cooking Time: Thirty minutes

Yields: 4 servings

Nutrition Facts: Calories: 154 | Carbs: 9g | Protein: 19g | Fat: 2g | Fiber: 12g

Ingredients:

- 160 grams of buckwheat or brown rice
- 100 grams of kale (spinach would also be a good alternative)
- 200 ml of water
- 400 ml of coconut milk
- 160 grams of red lentils
- Two teaspoons each of
  - Garam masala
  - Turmeric
- One bird's eye chili, deseeded and finely chopped (plus more if you want it extra hot)
- Two cms of ginger, grated
- Three cloves of garlic, crushed or grated
- One red onion (small), sliced
- One tablespoon of olive oil

Method:

1. Take a large, deep saucepan and add the olive oil in it. Add the sliced onion and cook it on low heat with the lid closed for about five minutes so that they get softened.

2. Add the chili, ginger, and garlic and cook it for another minute.

3. Add a splash of water along with the garam masala and turmeric and cook for another minute.

4. Next add the coconut milk, red lentils along with 200 ml of water. You can do this by filling the can of coconut milk halfway with water and adding it into the saucepan.

5. Combine everything together properly and let it cook over low heat for about twenty minutes. Keep the lid on and keep stirring occasionally. If the dhal starts to stick to the pan, add a little more water to it.

6. Add the kale after twenty minutes and stir properly and put the lid back on. Let it cook for another five minutes. (If you're using spinach instead, cook for an additional one to two minutes)

7. Add the buckwheat in a medium-sized saucepan about fifteen minutes before the curry is cooked.

8. Add lots of boiling water into the buckwheat and boil the water again— Cook for about ten minutes. If you prefer softer buckwheat, you can cook it for a little longer.

9. Drain the buckwheat using a sieve and serve along with the dhal.

Chicken Curry

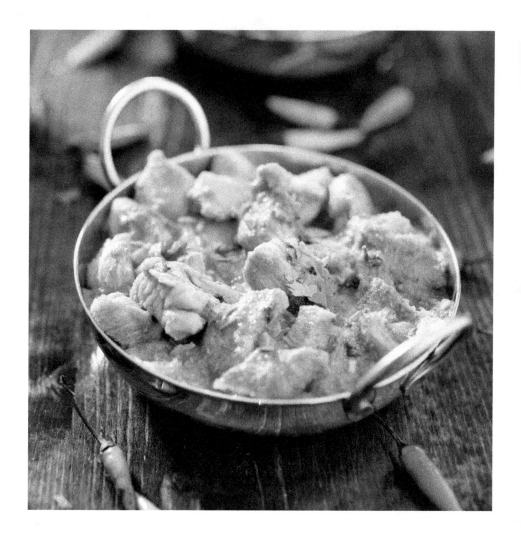

Total Prep & Cooking Time: 45 minutes

Yields: 4 servings

Nutrition Facts: Calories: 243 | Carbs: 7.5g | Protein: 28g | Fat: 11g | Fiber: 1.5g

Ingredients:

- 200 grams of buckwheat (you can also use basmati rice or brown rice)
- One 400ml tin of coconut milk
- Eight skinless and boneless chicken thighs, sliced into bite-sized chunks (you can also use four chicken breasts)
- One tablespoon of olive oil
- Six cardamom pods (optional)
- One cinnamon stick (optional)
- Two teaspoons each of
  - Ground turmeric
  - Ground cumin
  - Garam masala
- Two cm. of fresh ginger, peeled and coarsely chopped
- Three cloves of garlic, roughly chopped
- One red onion, roughly chopped
- Two tablespoons of freshly chopped coriander (and more for garnishing)

Method:

1. Add the ginger, garlic, and onions in a food processor and blitz to get a paste. You can also use a hand blender to make the paste. If you have neither, just finely chop the three ingredients and continue the following steps.

2. Add the turmeric powder, cumin, and garam masala into the paste and combine them together. Keep the paste aside.

3. Take a wide, deep pan (preferably a non-stick pan) and add one tablespoon of olive oil into it. Heat it over high heat for about a minute and then add the pieces of boneless chicken thighs. Increase the heat and stir-fry the chicken thighs for about two minutes. Then, reduce the heat and add the curry paste. Let the chicken cook in the curry paste for about three minutes and then pour half of the coconut milk (about 200ml) into it. You can also add the cardamom and cinnamon if you're using them.

4. Let it boil for some time and then reduce the heat and let it simmer for thirty minutes. The curry sauce will get thick and delicious.

5. You can add a splash of coconut milk if your curry sauce begins to get dry. You might not need to add extra coconut milk at all, but you can add it if you want a slightly more saucy curry.

6. Prepare your side dishes and other accompaniments (buckwheat or rice) while the curry is cooking.

7. Add the chopped coriander as a garnish when the curry is ready and serve immediately with the buckwheat or rice.

Chickpea Stew With Baked Potatoes

Total Prep & Cooking Time: One hour and ten minutes

Yields: 4 to 6 servings

Nutrition Facts: Calories: 348.3 | Carbs: 41.2g | Protein: 7.2g | Fat: 16.5g | Fiber: 5.3g

Ingredients:

- Two yellow peppers, chopped into bite-sized pieces (you can also use other colored bell peppers)
- Two 400-grams tins each of
  o Chickpeas (you can also use kidney beans) (don't drain the water if you prefer including it)
  o Chopped tomatoes
- Two cm. of ginger, grated
- Four cloves of garlic, crushed or grated
- Two red onions, finely chopped
- Four to six potatoes, prickled all over
- Two tablespoons each of
  o Turmeric
  o Cumin seeds
  o Olive oil
  o Unsweetened cocoa powder (or cacao, if you want)
  o Parsley (and extra for garnishing)

- Half a teaspoon to two teaspoons of chili flakes (you can add according to how hot you like things)
- A splash of water
- Side salad (optional)
- Salt and pepper according to your taste (optional)

Method:

1. Preheat your oven to 200 degrees Celsius.

2. In the meantime, prepare all the other ingredients.

3. Place your baking potatoes in the oven when it gets hot enough and allow it to cook for an hour so that they are cooked according to your preference. You can also use your regular method to bake the potatoes if it's different from this method.

4. When the potatoes are cooking in the oven, place a large wide saucepan over low heat and add the olive oil along with the chopped red onion into it. Keep the lid on and let the onions cook for five minutes. The onions should turn soft but shouldn't turn brown.

5. Take the lid off and add the chili, cumin, ginger, and garlic into the saucepan. Let it cook on low heat for another minute and then add the turmeric along with a tiny splash of water and cook it for a further minute. Make sure that the pan does not get too dry.

6. Then, add in the yellow pepper, canned chickpeas (along with the chickpea liquid), cacao or cocoa powder, and chopped tomatoes. Bring

the mixture to a boil and then let it simmer on low heat for about forty-five minutes so that the sauce gets thick and unctuous (make sure that it doesn't burn). The stew and the potatoes should complete cooking at roughly the same time.

7. Finally, add some salt and pepper as per your taste along with the parsley and stir them in the stew.

8. You can add the stew on top of the baked potatoes and serve. You can also serve the stew with a simple side salad.

Blueberry Pancakes

Total Prep & Cooking Time: 25 minutes

Yields: 2 servings

Nutrition Facts: Calories: 84 | Carbs: 11g | Protein: 2.3g | Fat: 3.5g | Fiber: 0g

Ingredients:

- 225 grams of blueberries
- 150 grams of rolled oats
- Six eggs
- Six bananas
- One-fourth of a teaspoon of salt
- Two teaspoons of baking powder

Method:

1. Add the rolled oats in a high-speed blender and pulse it for about a minute or so to get the oat flour. Before adding the oats to the blender, make sure that it is very dry. Otherwise, your oat flour will turn soggy.

2. Then, add the eggs and bananas along with the salt and baking soda into the blender and blend them together for another two minutes until you get a smooth batter.

3. Take a large bowl and transfer the mixture into it. Then add the blueberries and fold them into the mixture. Let it rest for about ten minutes to allow the baking powder to activate.

4. To make the pancakes, place a frying pan on medium-high heat and add a dollop of butter into it. The butter will help to make your pancakes really crispy and delicious.

5. Add a few spoonfuls of the blueberry pancake batter into the frying pan and cook it until the bottom side turns golden. Once the bottom turns golden, toss the pancake and fry the other side.

6. Serve them hot and enjoy.

Sirtfood Bites

Total Prep & Cooking Time: 1 hour + 15 minutes

Yields: 15-20 bites

Nutrition Facts: Calories: 58.1 | Carbs: 10.1g | Protein: 0.9g | Fat: 2.3g | Fiber: 1.2g

Ingredients:

- One tablespoon each of
  - Extra virgin olive oil
  - Ground turmeric
  - Cocoa powder
- Nine ounces of Medjool dates, pitted (about 250 grams)
- One ounce (about thirty grams) of dark chocolate (85% cocoa solids), break them into pieces (you can also use one-fourth of a cup of cocoa nibs)
- One teaspoon of vanilla extract (you can also take the scraped seeds of one vanilla pod)
- One cup of walnuts (about 120 grams)
- One to two tablespoons of water

Method:

1. Add the chocolate and walnuts in a food processor and blitz them until you get a fine powder.

2. Add the Medjool dates, cocoa powder, ground turmeric, extra-virgin olive oil, and vanilla extract into the food processor and blend them together until the mixture forms a ball. Depending on the consistency of the mixture, you can choose to add or skip the water. Make sure that the mixture is not too sticky.

3. Make bite-sized balls from the mixture using your hands and keep them in the refrigerator in an airtight container. Refrigerate them for at least an hour before consuming them.

4. To get a finish of your liking, you can roll the balls in some more dried coconut or cocoa. You can store the balls in the refrigerator for up to a week.

Flank Steak With Broccoli Cauliflower Gratin

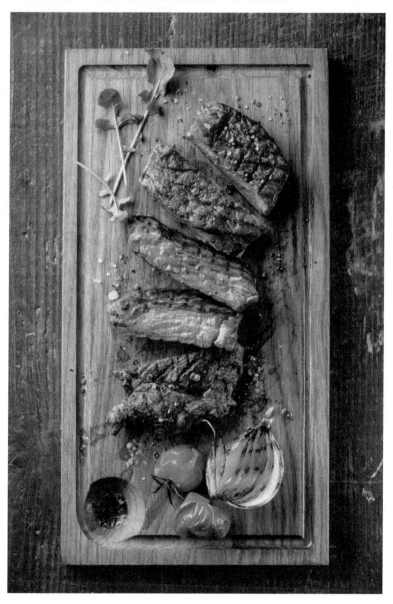

Total Prep & Cooking Time: 55 minutes

Yields: 4 servings

Nutrition Facts: Calories: 839 | Carbs: 8g | Protein: 43g | Fat: 70g | Fiber: 3g

Ingredients:

- Two tablespoons of olive oil
- Twenty ounces of flank steak
- One-fourth teaspoon salt
- Four ounces of divided shredded cheese
- Half cup of heavy whipping cream
- Eight ounces of cauliflower
- Eight ounces of broccoli
- Salt and pepper

For the pepper sauce,

- One tablespoon soy sauce
- One and a half cups of heavy whipping cream
- Half teaspoon ground black pepper

For the garnishing,

- Two tablespoons of freshly chopped parsley

Method:

1. At first, you have to preheat your oven to four hundred degrees Fahrenheit. Then you need to apply butter on a baking dish (eight by eight inches).

2. Then you have to clean and then trim the cauliflower and broccoli. Then you need to cut them into florets, and their stem needs to be sliced.

3. Then you have to boil the broccoli and cauliflower for about five minutes in salted water.

4. After boiling, you need to drain out all the water and keep the vegetables aside. Then you have to take a saucepan over medium heat and add half portion of the shredded cheese, heavy cream, and salt. Then you need to whisk them together until the cheese gets melted. Then you have to add the cauliflower and the broccoli and mix them in.

5. Place the cauliflower and broccoli mixture in a baking dish. Then you have to take the rest half portion of the cheese and add—Bake for about twenty minutes in the oven.

6. Season with salt and pepper on both sides of the meat.

7. Then you have to take a large frying pan over medium-high heat and fry the meat for about four to five minutes on each side.

8. After that, take a cutting board and place the meat on it. Then you have to leave the meat for about ten to fifteen minutes before you start to slice it.

9. Take the frying pan, and in it, you need to pour soy sauce, cream, and pepper. Then you have to bring it to a boil and allow the sauce to simmer until the sauce becomes creamy in texture. Then you need to taste it and then season it with some more salt and pepper according to your taste.

Kale Celery Salad

Total Prep & Cooking Time: 15 minutes

Yields: 4 servings

Nutrition Facts: 196 | Carbs: 20g | Protein: 5.7g | Fat: 11.5g | Fiber: 4.8g

Ingredients:

- Half a cup of crumbled feta cheese
- Half a cup of chopped and toasted walnuts
- One wedge lemon
- One red apple, crisp
- Two celery stalks
- Eight dates, pitted dried
- Four cups of washed and dried baby kale (stemmed)

For the dressing,

- Three tbsps. olive oil
- One tsp. maple syrup (or you can use any other sweetener as per your preference)
- Four tsps. balsamic vinegar
- Freshly ground salt and black pepper

Method:

1. At first, you have to take a platter or a wide serving bowl. Then you need to place the baby kale in it.

2. Cut the dates into very thin slices, lengthwise. Then you need to place it in another small bowl.

3. After that, you have to peel the celery and then cut them into halves, lengthwise.

4. Then you need to take your knife, hold it in a diagonal angle, and then cut the celery into thin pieces (approximately one to two inches each). Add these pieces to the dates.

5. Then you have to cut the sides off the apple. You need to cut very thin slices from those pieces.

6. Over the apple slices, you need to put some lemon juice to prevent them from browning.

7. For preparing the dressing, you have to take a small bowl, add maple syrup, olive oil, and vinegar. Then you need to whisk them together.

8. Once done, you have to season with freshly ground pepper and two pinches of salt.

9. Before serving, you need to take most of the dressing and pour it over the salad. Then you have to toss nicely so that they get combined. Then you need to pour the rest of the portion of the dressing over the dates and celery.

10. On the top, you have to add the date mixture, feta cheese, apple slices, and walnuts.

Buckwheat Stir Fry

Total Prep & Cooking Time: 28 minutes

Yields: 8 servings

Nutrition Facts: Calories: 258 | Carbs: 35.1g | Protein: 6.8g | Fat: 11.9g | Fiber: 2g

Ingredients:

For the buckwheat,

- Three cups of water
- One and a half cups of uncooked roasted buckwheat groats
- Pinch of salt

For the stir fry,

- Half a cup of finely chopped basil
- Half a cup of finely chopped parsley
- One teaspoon salt
- Four tablespoons of divided red palm oil or coconut oil
- Two cups of drained and chopped marinated artichoke hearts
- Four large bell peppers (sliced into strips)
- Four large minced cloves of garlic
- One bunch of finely chopped kale (ribs removed)

Method:

For making the buckwheat,

1. In a medium-sized pot, pour the buckwheat. Then rinse with cold water and drain the water. Repeat this process for about two to three times.

2. Then add three cups of water to it and also add a pinch of salt. Cover the pot and bring it to a boil.

3. Reduce the heat to low and then cook for about fifteen minutes. Keep the lid on and remove the pot from the heat.

4. Leave it for three minutes and then fluff with a fork.

For making the stir fry,

1. At first, you have to take a ceramic non-stick wok and preheat over medium heat. Then you need to add one tablespoon of oil and coat it. Then you have to add garlic and then sauté for about ten seconds. Then you need to add kale and then add one-fourth teaspoon of salt. Then you need to sauté it accompanied by occasional stirring, until it shrinks in half. Then you have to transfer it to a medium-sized bowl.

2. Then again return to the wok, turn the heat on high, and pour one tablespoon of oil. You need to add one-fourth teaspoon salt and pepper. Then you have to sauté it until it turns golden brown in color. Once done, you need to place it in the bowl containing kale.

3. Then you have to reduce the heat to low, and you need to add two tablespoons of oil. Add the cooked buckwheat and stir it nicely so that it gets coated in the oil. Then after turning off the heat, you need to add the kale and peppers, basil, parsley, artichoke hearts, and half teaspoon salt. Gently stir and serve it hot.

Kale Omelet

Total Prep & Cooking Time: 10 minutes

Yields: 1 serving

Nutrition Facts: Calories: 339 | Carbs: 8.6g | Protein: 15g | Fat: 28.1g | Fiber: 4.4g

Ingredients:

- One-fourth sliced avocado
- Pinch of red pepper (crushed)
- One tsp. sunflower seeds (unsalted)
- One tbsp. of freshly chopped cilantro
- One tbsp. lime juice
- One cup of chopped kale
- Two tsps. of extra-virgin olive oil
- One tsp. of low-fat milk
- Two eggs
- Salt

Method:

1. At first, take a small bowl and pour milk. Then you have to add the eggs and salt to it. Beat the mixture thoroughly. Then take a small non-stick

skillet over medium heat, and add one tsp. of oil and heat it. Then add the egg mixture and cook for about one to two minutes, until the time you notice that the center is still a bit runny, but the bottom has become set. Then you need to flip the omelet and cook the other side for another thirty seconds until it is set too. One done, transfer the omelet to a plate.

2. Toss the kale with one tsp. of oil, sunflower seeds, cilantro, lime juice, salt, and crushed red pepper in another bowl. Then return to the omelet on the plate and top it off with avocado and the kale salad.

Tuna Rocket Salad

Total Prep & Cooking Time: 20 minutes

Yields: 4 servings

Nutrition Facts: Calories: 321 | Carbs: 20g | Protein: 33g | Fat: 12g | Fiber: 9.5g

Ingredients:

- Twelve leaves of basil (fresh)
- Two bunches of washed and dried rocket (trimmed)
- One and a half tbsps. of olive oil
- Freshly ground black pepper and salt
- Sixty grams of kalamata olives cut into halves, lengthwise (drained pitted)
- One thinly sliced and halved red onion
- Two coarsely chopped ripe tomatoes
- Four hundred grams of rinsed and drained cannellini beans
- Four hundred grams of drained tuna
- 2 cm cubes of one multigrain bread roll

Method:

1. At first, you need to preheat your oven to 200 degrees Celsius.

2. After that, take a baking tray and line it with a foil.

3. Then you have to spread the cubes of bread over the baking tray evenly.

4. Put the baking tray inside the oven and cook it for about ten minutes until it turns golden in color.

5. In the meantime, you have to take a large bowl and add the olives, onions, tomatoes, cannellini beans, and tuna. Then you need to season it with pepper and salt. Add some oil and then toss for smooth combining.

6. Your next step is to add the basil leaves, croutons, and the rocket. Then you need to toss gently to combine. After that, you can divide the salad into the serving bowls and serve.

Turmeric Baked Salmon

Total Prep & Cooking Time: 30 minutes

Yields: 4 servings

Nutrition Facts: Calories: 448 | Carbs: 2g | Protein: 34g | Fat: 33g | Fiber: 0.2g

Ingredients:

- One ripe yellow lemon
- Half a teaspoon of salt
- One teaspoon turmeric
- One tablespoon of dried thyme
- Half a cup of frozen, salted butter (you may require some more for greasing the pan)
- Four fresh one and a half inches thick salmon fillets (skin-on)

Method:

1. At first, you need to preheat your oven to 400 degrees Fahrenheit. Then with a thin layer of butter, you need to grease the bottom of the baking sheet. Rinse the salmon fillets and pat them dry. Then you have to place the salmon fillets on the buttered baking dish keeping the skin side down.

2. Take the lemons and cut them into four round slices. Remove the seeds and then cut each slice into two halves. Then you will have eight pieces.

3. Take a small dish and combine turmeric, dried thyme, and salt. Then you need to mix them well until they are nicely combined. On the top of the salmon fillets, you need to evenly sprinkle the spice mixture.

4. Place two lemon slices over each salmon fillet.

5. After that, you need to grate the cold butter on the top of the salmon fillets evenly. Allow the butter to meltdown and form a delicious sauce.

6. Then you have to cover the pan with parchment or aluminum foil. Put it inside the oven and cook for about fifteen to twenty minutes according to your desire. The cooking time is dependent on the thickness of the salmon fillets. You can check whether it is done or not by cutting into the center.

7. Once done, remove it from the oven and then uncover it. The butter sauce needs to be spooned over from the tray.

8. Top it off with fresh mint and serve.

Chapter 4: One-Week Meal Plan

Day 1

8 AM – Green Juice

12 PM - Blueberry Kale Smoothie

4 PM – Tropical Kale Smoothie

8 PM – Turmeric Baked Salmon

Day 2

8 AM – Tropical Kale Smoothie

12 PM – Green Juice

4 PM – Strawberry Oatmeal Smoothie

8 PM – King Prawns and Buckwheat Noodles

Day 3

8 AM – Strawberry Oatmeal Smoothie

12 PM – Tropical Kale Smoothie

4 PM – Green Juice

8 PM – Buckwheat Stir Fry

Day 4

8 AM – Blueberry Kale Smoothie

12 PM – Green Juice

4 PM – Green Juice Salad

8 PM – Tuna Rocket Salad

Day 5

8 AM – Green Juice

12 PM – Tropical Kale Smoothie

4 PM – Sirtfood Bites

8 PM – Chicken Curry

Day 6

8 AM – Strawberry Oatmeal Smoothie

12 PM – Green Juice

4 PM – Kale Celery Salad

8 PM – Flank Steak with Broccoli Cauliflower Gratin

Day 7

8 AM – Tropical Kale Smoothie

12 PM – Blueberry Kale Smoothie

4 PM – Kale Omelet

8 PM – Chickpea Stew with Baked Potatoes

PART IV

In this chapter, we are going to study the details of the reset diet and what recipes you can make.

Chapter 1: How to Reset Your Body?

Created by a celebrity trainer, Harley Pasternak, the body reset diet is a famous fifteen-day eating pattern that aims to jump-start weight loss. According to Pasternak, if you experience rapid loss in weight early in a diet, you will feel more motivated to stick to that diet plan. This theory is even supported by a few scientific studies (Alice A Gibson, 2017).

The body reset diet claims to help in weight loss with light exercise and low-calorie diet plans for fifteen days. The diet is divided into 3 phases of five days each. Each phase had a particular pattern of diet and exercise routine. You need to consume food five times every day, starting from the first phase, which mostly consists of smoothies and progressing to more solid foods in the second and third phases.

The three phases of the body reset diet are:

- **Phase One** – During this stage, you are required to consume only two snacks every day and drink smoothies for breakfast, lunch, and dinner. In the case of exercise, you have to walk at least ten thousand steps per day.

- **Phase Two** – During this phase, you can eat two snacks each day, consume solid food only once, and have to replace any two meals of the day with smoothies. In case of exercise, apart from walking ten thousand steps every day, on three of the days, you also have to finish five minutes of resistance training with the help of four separate exercises.

- **Phase Three** – You can consume two snacks every day, but you have to eat two low-calorie meals and replace one of your meals with a smoothie. For exercise, you are required to walk ten thousand steps. Apart from that, you also have to finish five minutes of resistance training with the help of four separate exercises each day.

After you have finished the standard fifteen-day diet requirements, you have to keep following the meal plan you followed in the third phase. However, during this time, you are allowed to have two "free meals" twice a week in which you can consume anything you want. These "free meals" are meant as a reward so that you can avoid feeling deprived. According to Pasternak, depriving yourself of a particular food continuously can result in binge eating (Nawal Alajmi, 2016).

There is no official endpoint of the diet after the first fifteen days for losing and maintaining weight. Pasternak suggests that the habits and routines formed over fifteen days should be maintained for a lifetime.

Chapter 2: Science Behind Metabolism Reset

Several people take on a "cleanse" or "detox" diet every year to lose the extra holiday weight or simply start following healthy habits. However, some fat diet plans are often a bit overwhelming. For example, it requires a tremendous amount of self-discipline to drink only juices. Moreover, even after finishing a grueling detox diet plan, you might just go back to eating foods that are bad for you because of those days of deprivation. New studies issued in the *Medicine & Science in Sports & Exercise* shows that low-calorie diets may result in binge eating, which is not the right method for lasting weight loss.

Another research conducted by the researchers at Loughborough University showed that healthy, college-aged women who followed a calorie-restricted diet consumed an extra three hundred calories at dinner as compared to the control group who consumed three standard meals. They revealed that it was because they had lower levels of peptide YY (represses appetite) and higher levels of ghrelin (makes you hungry). They are most likely to go hog wild when you are feeling ravenous, and it's finally time to eat (Nawal Alajmi K. D.-O., 2016).

Another research published in *Cognitive Neuroscience* studied the brains of chronic dieters. They revealed that there was a weaker connection between the two regions of the brain in people who had a higher percentage of body fat. They showed that they might have an increased risk of getting obese because it's harder for them to set their temptations aside (Pin-Hao Andy Chen, 2016).

A few other studies, however, also revealed that you could increase your self-control through practice. Self-control, similar to any other kind of strength, also requires time to develop. However, you can consider focusing on a diet plan that can help you "reset" instead of putting all your efforts into developing your self-control to get healthy.

A reset is considered as a new start – one that can get your metabolism and your liver in good shape. The liver is the biggest solid organ of your body, and it's mainly responsible for removing toxins that can harm your health and well-being by polluting your system. Toxins keep accumulating in your body all the time, and even though it's the liver's job to handle this, it can sometimes get behind schedule, which can result in inflammation. It causes a lot of strain on your metabolism and results in weight gain, particularly around the abdomen. The best method to alleviate this inflammation is to follow a metabolism rest diet and give your digestive system a vacation (Olivia M. Farr, 2015).

Chapter 3: Recipes for Smoothies and Salads

If you want to lose weight and you have a particular period within which you want to achieve it, then here are some recipes that are going to be helpful.

Green Smoothie

Total Prep & Cooking Time: 2 minutes

Yields: 1 serving

Nutrition Facts: Calories: 144 | Carbs: 28.2g | Protein: 3.4g | Fat: 2.9g | Fiber: 4.8g

Ingredients:

- One cup each of
  - Almond milk
  - Raw spinach
- One-third of a cup of strawberries
- One orange, peeled

Method:

1. Add the peeled orange, strawberries, almond milk, and raw spinach in a blender and blend everything until you get a smooth paste. You can add extra water if required to achieve the desired thickness.

2. Pour out the smoothie into a glass and serve.

Strawberry Banana Smoothie

Total Prep & Cooking Time: 5 minutes

Yields: 2 servings

Nutrition Facts: Calories: 198| Carbs: 30.8g | Protein: 5.9g | Fat: 7.1g | Fiber: 4.8g

Ingredients:

- Half a cup each of
  - Milk
  - Greek yogurt
- One banana, frozen and quartered
- Two cups of fresh strawberries, halved

Method:

1. Add the milk, Greek yogurt, banana, and strawberries into a high-powered blender and blend until you get a smooth mixture.

2. Pour the smoothie equally into two separate glasses and serve.

Notes:

- *Don't add ice to the smoothie as it can make it watery very quickly. Using frozen bananas will keep your smoothie cold.*

- *As you're using bananas and strawberries, there is no need to add any artificial sweetener.*

Salmon Citrus Salad

Total Prep & Cooking Time: 20 minutes

Yields: 6 servings

Nutrition Facts: Calories: 336 | Carbs: 20g | Protein: 17g | Fat: 21g | Fiber: 5g

Ingredients:

- One pound of Citrus Salmon (slow-roasted)
- Half of an English cucumber, sliced
- One tomato (large), sliced into a quarter of an inch thick pieces
- One grapefruit, peeled and cut into segments
- Two oranges, peeled and cut into segments
- Three beets, roasted and quartered
- One avocado
- Boston lettuce leaves
- Two tablespoons of red wine vinegar
- Half of a red onion
- Flakey salt
- Aleppo pepper flakes

For the Citrus Shallot Vinaigrette,

- Five tablespoons of olive oil (extra-virgin)
- One clove of garlic, smashed
- Salt and pepper
- One and a half tablespoons of rice wine vinegar
- Two tablespoons of orange juice or fresh lemon juice

- One tablespoon of shallot, minced

Method:

For preparing the Citrus Shallot Vinaigrette:

1. Add the ingredients for the vinaigrette in a bowl and whisk them together.

2. Keep the mixture aside.

For assembling the salad,

1. Add the onions and vinegar in a small bowl and pickle them by letting them sit for about fifteen minutes.

2. In the meantime, place the lettuce leaves on the serving plate.

3. Dice the avocado in half and eliminate the pit. Then scoop the flesh and add them onto the plate. Sprinkle a dash of flakey salt and Aleppo pepper on top to season it.

4. Add the quartered beets onto the serving plate along with the grapefruit and orange segments.

5. Salt the cucumber and tomato slices lightly and add them onto the plate.

6. Then, scatter the pickled onions on top and cut the salmon into bits and add it on the plate.

7. Lastly, drizzle the Citrus Shallot Vinaigrette on top of the salad and finish off with a dash of flakey salt.

Chapter 4: Quick and Easy Breakfast and Main Course Recipes

Quinoa Salad

Total Prep & Cooking Time: 40 minutes

Yields: Eight servings

Nutrition Facts: Calories: 205 | Carbs: 25.9g | Protein: 6.1g | Fat: 9.4g | Fiber: 4.6g

Ingredients:

- One tablespoon of red wine vinegar
- One-fourth of a cup each of
    o Lemon juice (about two to three lemons)
    o Olive oil
- One cup each of
    o Quinoa (uncooked), rinsed with the help of a fine-mesh colander
    o Flat-leaf parsley (from a single large bunch), finely chopped
- Three-fourth of a cup of red onion (one small red onion), chopped
- One red bell pepper (medium-sized), chopped
- One cucumber (medium-sized), seeded and chopped
- One and a half cups of chickpeas (cooked), or One can of chickpeas (about fifteen ounces), rinsed and drained
- Two cloves of garlic, minced or pressed
- Two cups of water
- Black pepper, freshly ground
- Half a teaspoon of fine sea salt

Method:

1. Place a medium-sized saucepan over medium-high heat and add the rinsed quinoa into it along with the water. Allow the mixture to boil and then reduce the heat and simmer it. Cook for about fifteen minutes so that the quinoa has absorbed all the water. As time goes on, decrease the heat and maintain a gentle simmer. Take the saucepan away from the heat and cover it with a lid. Allow the cooked quinoa to rest for about five minutes to give it some time to increase in size.

2. Add the onions, bell pepper, cucumber, chickpeas, and parsley in a large serving bowl and mix them together. Keep the mixture aside.

3. Add the garlic, vinegar, lemon juice, olive oil, and salt in another small bowl and whisk the ingredients so that they are appropriately combined. Keep this mixture aside.

4. When the cooked quinoa has almost cooled down, transfer it to the serving bowl. Add the dressing on top and toss to combine everything together.

5. Add an extra pinch of sea salt and the black pepper to season according to your preference. Allow the salad to rest for five to ten minutes before serving it for the best results.

6. You can keep the salad in the refrigerator for up to four days. Make sure to cover it properly.

7. You can serve it at room temperature or chilled.

Notes: Instead of cooking additional quinoa, you can use about three cups of leftover quinoa for making this salad. Moreover, you can also serve this salad with fresh greens and an additional drizzle of lemon juice and olive oil. You can also add a dollop of cashew sour cream or crumbled feta cheese as a topping.

Herb and Goat Cheese Omelet

Total Prep & Cooking Time: 20 minutes

Yields: Two servings

Nutrition Facts: Calories: 233 | Carbs: 3.6g | Protein: 16g | Fat: 17.6g | Fiber: 1g

Ingredients:

- Half a cup each of
  - Red bell peppers (3 x quarter-inch), julienne-cut
  - Zucchini, thinly sliced
- Four large eggs
- Two teaspoons of olive oil, divided
- One-fourth of a cup of goat cheese (one ounce), crumbled
- Half a teaspoon of fresh tarragon, chopped
- One teaspoon each of
  - Fresh parsley, chopped
  - Fresh chives, chopped
- One-eighth of a teaspoon of salt
- One-fourth of a teaspoon of black pepper, freshly ground (divided)
- One tablespoon of water

Method:

1. Break the eggs into a bowl and add one tablespoon of water into it. Whisk them together and add in one-eighth of a teaspoon each of salt and ground black pepper.

2. In another small bowl, mix the goat cheese, tarragon, and parsley and keep it aside.

3. Place a nonstick skillet over medium heat and heat one teaspoon of olive oil in it. Add in the sliced zucchini, bell pepper, and the remaining one-eighth of a teaspoon of black pepper along with a dash of salt. Cook for about four minutes so that the bell pepper and zucchini get soft. Transfer the zucchini-bell pepper mixture onto a plate and cover it with a lid to keep it warm.

4. Add about half a teaspoon of oil into a skillet and add in half of the whisked egg into it. Do not stir the eggs and let the egg set slightly. Loosen the set edges of the omelet carefully with the help of a spatula. Tilt the skillet to move the uncooked part of the egg to the side. Keep following this method for about five seconds so that there is no more runny egg in the skillet. Add half of the crumbled goat cheese mixture evenly over the omelet and let it cook for another minute so that it sets.

5. Transfer the omelet onto a plate and fold it into thirds.

6. Repeat the process with the rest of the egg mixture, half a teaspoon of olive oil, and the goat cheese mixture.

7. Add the chopped chives on top of the omelets and serve with the bell pepper and zucchini mixture.

Mediterranean Cod

Total Prep & Cooking Time: 15 minutes

Yields: 4 servings

Nutrition Facts: Calories: 320 | Carbs: 31g | Protein: 35g | Fat: 8g | Fiber: 8g

Ingredients:

- One pound of spinach
- Four fillets of cod (almost one and a half pounds)
- Two zucchinis (medium-sized), chopped
- One cup of marinara sauce
- One-fourth of a teaspoon of red pepper, crushed
- Two cloves of garlic, chopped
- One tablespoon of olive oil
- Salt and pepper, according to taste
- Whole wheat roll, for serving

Method:

1. Place a ten-inch skillet on medium heat and add the marinara sauce and zucchini into it. Combine them together and let it simmer on medium heat.

2. Add the fillets of cod into the simmering sauce. Add one-fourth of a teaspoon each of salt and pepper too. Cover the skillet with a lid and let it cook for about seven minutes so that the cod gets just opaque throughout.

3. In the meantime, place a five-quart saucepot on medium heat and heat the olive oil in it. Add in the crushed red pepper and minced garlic. Stir and cook for about a minute.

4. Then, add in the spinach along with one-eighth of a teaspoon of salt. Cover the saucepot with a lid and let it cook for about five minutes, occasionally stirring so that the spinach gets wilted.

5. Add the spinach on the plates and top with the sauce and cod mixture and serve with the whole wheat roll.

Grilled Chicken and Veggies

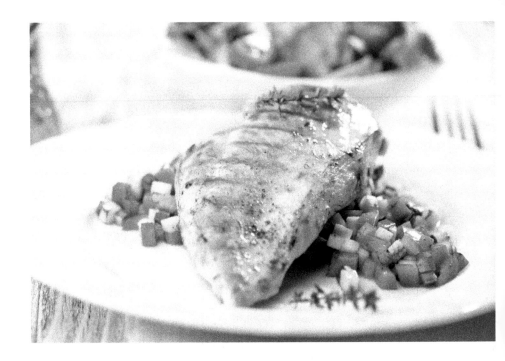

Total Prep & Cooking Time: 35 minutes

Yields: 4 servings

Nutrition Facts: Calories: 305 | Carbs: 11g | Protein: 26g | Fat: 17g | Fiber: 3g

Ingredients:

For the marinade,

- Four cloves of garlic, crushed
- One-fourth of a cup each of
  - Fresh lemon juice
  - Olive oil
- One teaspoon each of
  - Salt
  - Smoked paprika
  - Dried oregano
- Black pepper, according to taste
- Half a teaspoon of red chili flakes

For the grilling,

- Two to three zucchinis or courgette (large), cut into thin slices
- Twelve to sixteen spears of asparagus, woody sides trimmed
- Broccoli
- Two bell peppers, seeds eliminated and cut into thin slices
- Four pieces of chicken breasts (large), skinless and de-boned

Method:

1. Preheat your griddle or grill pan.

2. Sprinkle some salt on top of the chicken breasts to season them. Keep them aside to rest while you prepare the marinade.

3. For the marinade, mix all the ingredients properly.

4. Add about half of the marinade over the vegetables and the other half over the seasoned chicken breasts. Allow the marinade to rest for a couple of minutes.

5. Place the chicken pieces on the preheated grill. Grill for about five to seven minutes on each side until they are cooked according to your preference. The time on the grill depends on the thickness of the chicken breasts.

6. Remove them from the grill and cover them using a foil. Set it aside to rest and prepare to grill the vegetables in the meantime.

7. Grill the vegetables for a few minutes until they begin to char and are crispy yet tender.

8. Remove them from the grill and transfer them onto a serving plate. Serve the veggies along with the grilled chicken and add the lemon wedges on the side for squeezing.

Notes: You can add as much or as little vegetables as you like. The vegetable amounts are given only as a guide. Moreover, feel free to replace some of them with the vegetables you like to eat.

Stuffed Peppers

Total Prep & Cooking Time: 50 minutes

Yields: 4 servings

Nutrition Facts: Calories: 438 | Carbs: 32g | Protein: 32g | Fat: 20g | Fiber: 5g

Ingredients:

For the stuffed peppers,

- One pound of ground chicken or turkey
- Four bell peppers (large) of any color
- One and a quarter of a cups of cheese, shredded
- One and a half cups of brown rice, cooked (you can use cauliflower rice or quinoa)
- One can (about fourteen ounces) of fire-roasted diced tomatoes along with its juices
- Two teaspoons of olive oil (extra-virgin)
- One teaspoon each of
  - Garlic powder
  - Ground cumin
- One tablespoon of ground chili powder
- One-fourth of a teaspoon of black pepper
- Half a teaspoon of kosher salt

For serving,

- Sour cream or Greek yogurt

- Salsa

- Freshly chopped cilantro

- Avocado, sliced

- Freshly squeezed lemon juice

Method:

1. Preheat your oven to 375 degrees Fahrenheit.

2. Take a nine by thirteen-inch baking dish and coat it lightly with a nonstick cooking spray.

3. Take the bell peppers and slice them from top to bottom into halves. Remove the membranes and the seeds. Keep the bell peppers in the baking dish with the cut-side facing upwards.

4. Place a large, nonstick skillet on medium-high heat and heat the olive oil in it. Add in the chicken, pepper, salt, garlic powder, ground cumin, and chili powder and cook for about four minutes so that the chicken is cooked through and gets brown. Break apart the chicken while it's cooking. Drain off any excess liquid and then add in the can of diced tomatoes along with the juices. Allow it to simmer for a minute.

5. Take the pan away from the heat. Add in the cooked rice along with three-fourth of a cup of the shredded cheese and stir everything together.

6. Add this filling inside the peppers and add the remaining shredded cheese as a topping.

7. Add a little amount of water into the pan containing the peppers so that it barely covers the bottom of the pan.

8. Keep it uncovered and bake it in the oven for twenty-five to thirty-five minutes so that the cheese gets melted and the peppers get soft.

9. Add any of your favorite fixings as a topping and serve hot.

Notes:

- *For preparing the stuffed peppers ahead of time, make sure to allow the rice and chicken mixture to cool down completely before filling the peppers. You can prepare the stuffed peppers before time, and then you have to cover it with a lid and keep it in the refrigerator for a maximum of twenty-four hours before baking the peppers.*

- *If you're planning to reheat the stuffed peppers, gently reheat them in your oven or microwave. If you're using a microwave for this purpose, make sure to cut the peppers into pieces to warm them evenly.*

- *You can store any leftovers in the freezer for up to three months. Alternatively, you can keep them in the refrigerator for up to four days. Allow it to thaw in the fridge overnight.*

Brussels Sprouts With Honey Mustard Chicken

Total Prep & Cooking Time: Fifty minutes

Yields: Four servings

Nutrition Facts: Calories: 360 | Carbs: 14.5g | Protein: 30.8g | Fat: 20g | Fiber: 3.7g

Ingredients:

- One and a half pounds of Brussels sprouts, divided into two halves
- Two pounds of chicken thighs, skin-on and bone-in (about four medium-sized thighs)
- Three cloves of garlic, minced
- One-fourth of a large onion, cut into slices
- One tablespoon each of
  o Honey
  o Whole-grain mustard
  o Dijon mustard
- Two tablespoons of freshly squeezed lemon juice (one lemon)
- One-fourth of a cup plus two tablespoons of olive oil (extra-virgin)
- Freshly ground black pepper
- Kosher salt
- Non-stick cooking spray

Method:

1. Preheat your oven to 425 degrees Fahrenheit.

2. Take a large baking sheet and grease it with nonstick cooking spray. Keep it aside.

3. Add the minced garlic, honey, whole-grain mustard, Dijon mustard, one tablespoon of the lemon juice, one-fourth cup of the olive oil in a medium-sized bowl and mix them together. Add the Kosher salt and black pepper to season according to your preference.

4. Dip the chicken thighs into the sauce with the help of tongs and coat both sides. Transfer the things on the baking sheet. You can get rid of any extra sauce.

5. Mix the red onion and Brussels sprouts in a medium-sized bowl and drizzle one tablespoon of lemon juice along with the remaining two tablespoons of olive oil onto it. Toss everything together until the vegetables are adequately coated.

6. Place the red onion-Brussels sprouts mixture on the baking sheet around the chicken pieces. Ensure that the chicken and vegetables are not overlapping.

7. Sprinkle a little amount of salt and pepper on the top and keep it in the oven to roast for about thirty to thirty-five minutes so that the Brussels sprouts get crispy and the chicken has an internal temperature of 165 degrees Fahrenheit and has turned golden brown.

8. Serve hot.

Quinoa Stuffed Chicken

Total Prep & Cooking Time: 50 minutes

Yields: Four servings

Nutrition Facts: Calories: 355 | Carbs: 28g | Protein: 30g | Fat: 13g | Fiber: 4g

Ingredients:

- One and a half cups of chicken broth
- Three-fourths of a cup of quinoa (any color of your choice)
- Four chicken breasts (boneless and skinless)
- One lime, zested and one tablespoon of lime juice
- One-fourth of a cup of cilantro, chipped
- One-third of a cup of unsweetened coconut, shaved or coconut chips
- One Serrano pepper, seeded and diced
- Two cloves of garlic, minced
- Half a cup of red onion, diced
- Three-fourth of a cup of bell pepper, diced
- One tablespoon of coconut oil
- One teaspoon each of
  - Salt
  - Chili powder
  - Ground cumin

Method:

1. Preheat your oven to 375 degrees Fahrenheit.

2. Take a rimmed baking sheet and line it with parchment paper.

3. Place a medium-sized saucepan over medium-high heat and add the coconut oil in it. After it has melted, add in the Serrano peppers, garlic, red onion, and bell pepper and sauté for about one to two minutes so that they soften just a bit. Make sure that the vegetables are still bright in color. Then transfer the cooked vegetables into a bowl.

4. Add the quinoa in the empty sauce pot and increase the heat to high. Pour the chicken broth in it along with half a teaspoon of salt. Close the lid of the pot and bring it to a boil, allowing the quinoa to cook for about fifteen minutes so that the surface of the quinoa develops vent holes, and the broth has absorbed completely. Take the pot away from the heat and allow it to steam for an additional five minutes.

5. In the meantime, cut a slit along the long side in each chicken breast. It will be easier with the help of a boning knife. You are making a deep pocket in each breast, having a half-inch border around the remaining three attached sides. Keep the knife parallel to the cutting board and cut through the middle of the breast and leaving the opposite side attached. Try to cut it evenly as it's challenging to cook thick uncut portions properly in the oven. After that, add salt, cumin, and chili powder on all sides of the chicken.

6. When the quinoa has turned fluffy, add in the lime juice, lime zest, shaved coconut, and sautéed vegetables and stir them in. Taste the mixture and adjust the salt as per your preference.

7. Add the confetti quinoa mixture inside the cavity of the chicken breast. Place the stuffed breasts on the baking sheet with the quinoa facing upwards. They'll look like open envelopes.

8. Bake them in the oven for about twenty minutes.

9. Serve warm.

Kale and Sweet Potato Frittata

Total Prep & Cooking Time: 30 minutes

Yields: 4 servings

Nutrition Facts: Calories: 144 | Carbs: 10g | Protein: 7g | Fat: 9g | Fiber: 2g

Ingredients:

- Three ounces of goat cheese
- Two cloves of garlic
- Half of a red onion (small)
- Two cups each of
    o   Sweet potatoes
    o   Firmly packed kale, chopped
- Two tablespoons of olive oil
- One cup of half-and-half
- Six large eggs
- Half a teaspoon of pepper, freshly ground
- One teaspoon of Kosher salt

Method:

1.   Preheat your oven to 350 degrees Fahrenheit.

2.   Add the eggs, half-and-half, salt, and black pepper in a bowl and whisk everything together.

3. Place a ten-inch ovenproof nonstick skillet over medium heat and add one tablespoon of oil in it. Sauté the sweet potatoes in the skillet for about eight to ten minutes so that they turn soft and golden brown. Transfer them onto a plate and keep warm.

4. Next, add in the remaining one tablespoon of oil and sauté the kale along with the red onions and garlic in it for about three to four minutes so that the kale gets soft and wilted. Then, add in the whisked egg mixture evenly over the vegetables and cook for an additional three minutes.

5. Add some goat cheese on the top and bake it in the oven for ten to fourteen minutes so that it sets.

Walnut, Ginger, and Pineapple Oatmeal

Total Prep & Cooking Time: 30 minutes

Yields: 4 servings

Nutrition Facts: Calories: 323 | Carbs: 61g | Protein: 6g | Fat: 8g | Fiber: 5g

Ingredients:

- Two large eggs
- Two cups each of
  o Fresh pineapple, coarsely chopped
  o Old-fashioned rolled oats
  o Whole milk

- One cup of walnuts, chopped
- Half a cup of maple syrup
- One piece of ginger
- Two teaspoons of vanilla extract
- Half a teaspoon of salt

Method:

1. Preheat your oven to 400 degrees Fahrenheit.

2. Add the ginger, walnuts, pineapple, oats, and salt in a large bowl and mix them together. Add the mixture evenly among four ten-ounce ramekins and keep them aside.

3. Whisk the eggs along with the milk, maple syrup, and vanilla extract in a medium-sized bowl. Pour one-quarter of this mixture into each ramekin containing the oat-pineapple mixture.

4. Keep the ramekins on the baking sheet and bake them in the oven for about twenty-five minutes until the oats turn light golden brown on the top and have set properly.

5. Serve with some additional maple syrup on the side.

Caprese Salad

Total Prep & Cooking Time: 15 minutes

Yields: 4 servings

Nutrition Facts: Calories: 216 | Carbs: 4g | Protein: 13g | Fat: 16g | Fiber: 1g

Ingredients:

For the salad,

- Nine basil leaves (medium-sized)
- Eight ounces of fresh whole-milk mozzarella cheese
- Two tomatoes (medium-sized)
- One-fourth of a teaspoon of black pepper, freshly ground
- Half a teaspoon of Kosher salt, or one-fourth of a teaspoon of sea salt

For the dressing,

- One teaspoon of Dijon mustard
- One tablespoon each of
  o Balsamic vinegar
  o Olive oil

Method:

1. Add the olive oil, balsamic vinegar, and Dijon mustard into a small bowl and whisk them together with the help of a small hand whisk so that you get a smooth salad dressing. Keep it aside.

2. Cut the tomatoes into thin slices and try to get ten slices in total.

3. Cut the mozzarella into nine thin slices with the help of a sharp knife.

4. Place the slices of tomatoes and mozzarella on a serving plate, alternating and overlapping one another. Then, add the basil leaves on the top.

5. Season the salad with black pepper and salt and drizzle the prepared dressing on top.

6. Serve immediately.

One-Pot Chicken Soup

Total Prep & Cooking Time: 30 minutes

Yields: 6 servings

Nutrition Facts: Calories: 201 | Carbs: 20g | Protein: 16g | Fat: 7g | Fiber: 16g

Ingredients:

- Three cups of loosely packed chopped kale (or other greens of your choice)
- Two cups of chicken, shredded
- One can of white beans (about fifteen ounces), slightly drained
- Eight cups of broth (vegetable broth or chicken broth)
- Four cloves of garlic, minced
- One cup of yellow or white onion, diced
- One tablespoon of avocado oil (skip if you are using bacon)
- One strip of uncured bacon, chopped (optional)
- Black pepper + sea salt, according to taste

Method:

1. Place a Dutch oven or a large pot over medium heat. When it gets hot, add in the oil or bacon (optional), stirring occasionally, and allow it to get hot for about a minute.

2. Then, add in the diced onion and sauté for four to five minutes, occasionally stirring so that the onions get fragrant and translucent. Add in the minced garlic next and sauté for another two to three minutes. Be careful so as not to burn the ingredients.

3. Then, add the chicken, slightly drained white beans, and broth and bring the mixture to a simmer. Cook for about ten minutes to bring out all the flavors. Taste the mixture and add salt and pepper to season according to your preference. Add in the chopped kale in the last few minutes of cooking. Cover the pot and let it cook until the kale has wilted.

4. Serve hot.

Notes: *You can store any leftovers in the freezer for up to a month. Or, you can store them in the refrigerator for a maximum of three to four days. Simply reheat on the stovetop or in the microwave and eat it later.*

Chocolate Pomegranate Truffles

Total Prep & Cooking Time: 10 minutes

Yields: Twelve to Fourteen truffles

Nutrition Facts: Calories: 95 | Carbs: 26g | Protein: 1g | Fat: 2g | Fiber: 3g

Ingredients:

- One-third of a cup of pomegranate arils
- Half a teaspoon each of
  o Vanilla extract
  o Ground cinnamon
- Half a cup of ground flax seed
- Two tablespoons of cocoa powder (unsweetened)
- About one tablespoon of water
- One and a half cups of pitted Medjool dates
- One-eighth of a teaspoon of salt

Method:

1. Add the pitted dates in a food processor and blend until it begins to form a ball. Add some water and pulse again. Add in the vanilla, cinnamon, flax seeds, cocoa powder, and salt and blend until everything is combined properly.

2. Turn off the food processor and unplug it. Add in the pomegranate arils and fold them in the mixture so that they are distributed evenly.

3. Make twelve to fourteen balls using the mixture. You can create an outer coating or topping if you want by rolling the balls in finely shredded coconut or cocoa powder.

Notes: You can store the chocolate pomegranate truffles in the fridge in an air-tight container for a maximum of three days.

PART V

Chapter 1: Noodles - Rice & Soup

Drunkard's Noodles

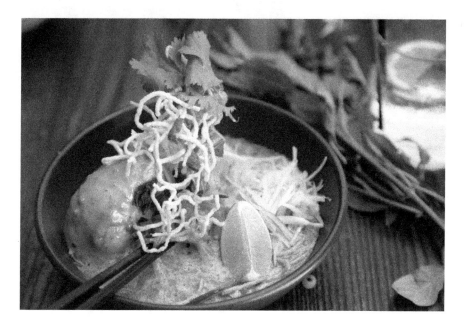

Servings Provided: 1-2

Time Required: 15 minutes

What is Needed:

- Wide rice noodles- prepared dry noodles (About 2 cups)
- Chicken meat/pork loin (.5 cup - chicken breast)
- Baby corn (1-2)
- Carrots (2 -3 small)
- Thai long chili - mild - yellow/red/orange (2-3 thin slivers)
- Fresh green peppercorns (1 bunch - leave the corns in the bunch)
- Finger root (10 tiny flakes/one average finger - cut into slivers)
- Thai hot chili (3-4 - whole red & green)
- Brown/yellow onion (half a slice)

- Garlic - not peeled (3-4 cloves)
- Thai Sweet Basil/Star of siam basil (1 cup)
- Dark sweet soy sauce (.5 tsp.)
- Oyster sauce (2 tsp.)
- White cane sugar (1 tbsp.)
- Light soy sauce (2 tsp.)

Preparation Method:

1. Fry the garlic, chili, and onions in oil for about one minute.
2. Cut the carrot lengthwise into slices. Mix in the corn, carrots, sweet chili, and green peppercorn bunch. Stir and simmer for another 10-15 seconds.
3. Slice and mix in the chicken and cook until nearly done, and add the soy sauce, sugar, and oyster sauce. Simmer until the sugar dissolves.
4. Add the pre-cooked rice noodles, coating them with the sauces.
5. Transfer the pan to a cool burner and garnish it with the fresh basil. Serve and enjoy it promptly.

Jasmine Rice

Servings Provided: 4-6

Time Required: 20 minutes

What is Needed:

- Water (2.75 cups + as needed)
- Jasmine rice (1.5 cups)
- Salt (.75 tsp.)

Preparation Method:

1. Boil the water with the salt. Stir in the rice, put a lid on the pot, and adjust the temperature setting to low. Let it simmer until all of the water is absorbed (15 min.).

2. Taste test the rice. Add a few tablespoons of water if it's too firm. Cover the pan and let the rice absorb the water.

Chicken Wonton Soup - Kiao Nam Gai

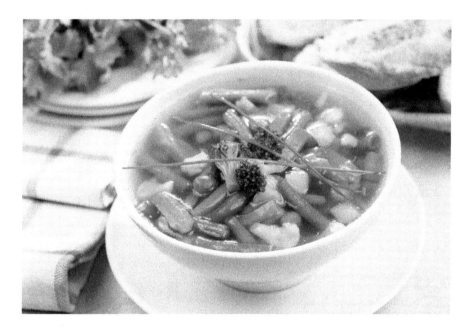

Servings Provided: 6-10

Time Required: Less than 45 minutes

What is Needed:

The Wontons:

- Ground chicken or pork (400 grams/about 14 oz.)
- Lemongrass (1 tsp.)
- Kaffir lime leaves (1 tsp.)
- Coriander Root (1 tsp.)
- Green onion (1 tsp.)
- Garlic (1 tsp.)
- Tapioca Starch (1 tsp.)
- White pepper - finely ground (1 tsp.)
- Sesame oil (.5 tsp.)
- Fish Sauce (.5 tsp.)
- Wonton wrappers (50)

The Broth:

- Chicken or vegetable stock (6-8 cups)
- Coriander root (1 tsp.)
- Garlic (1 tsp.)
- Oyster sauce (2 tsp.)
- Light soy sauce (1 tsp.)
- Sugar (1 tsp.)
- White pepper (.5 tsp.)
- Chinese cabbage/Bok Choy Leaves (4 - 6 heads)

Preparation Method:

1. Grind the kaffir lime leaf, lemongrass, garlic, and coriander root into a

smooth paste. Blend the mixture with the chopped meat, tapioca flour, green onion, white pepper, fish sauce, and sesame oil.

2. Fill and wrap the wontons.

3. Prepare the soup broth by adding white pepper, garlic, coriander root, oyster sauce, and soy sauce to the unseasoned chicken or vegetable stock. Boil hard for about five minutes.

4. In another soup pot, warm water and boil the wontons for about five minutes. Remove them and place them in a serving bowl.

5. Blanch the bok choy leaves for about one minute and place them in your bowls with the wontons.

6. Spoon enough of the broth over the bowl to cover the wontons and bok choy lightly.

7. Garnish them using chopped green onions and a bit of white pepper.

8. Serve with condiments, including sun-dried pickled green chilies, red chili flakes, sugar, and fish sauce with red chili.

Herbal Chicken Soup With Bitter Melon

Servings Provided: 4

Time Required: Less than 15 minutes

What is Needed:

- Breast portion chicken (half of 1)
- Bitter melon/Chinese bitter gourd (half of 1)
- Cilantro/Coriander leaves - roots attached (3-4)
- Galangal root (1-2-inch piece)
- Lemongrass (1 stalk)
- Thai hot chilies (2 or more)
- Garlic (2-3 cloves)
- Sugar (1 tsp.)
- Light soy sauce (1 tbsp.)
- Coconut/vegetable oil (1 tbsp.)

Preparation Method:

1. Discard the skin and chop the chicken into small cubes. Remove the seeds and inner pulp from the bitter melon and cut it also.
2. Dice the coriander and grind the garlic, red chili, and galangal into a rough pulp.
3. Prepare a skillet of coconut oil to fry the herbs for about half a minute and add the chicken to fry until cooked - slowly.
4. Pour in water and wait for it to boil.
5. Add the diced melon and simmer until tender (8 min.). Extinguish the heat and toss in the chopped coriander leaves.
6. Serve the soup while it's hot with a sprinkle of chopped coriander just before serving.

Pumpkin Coconut Soup

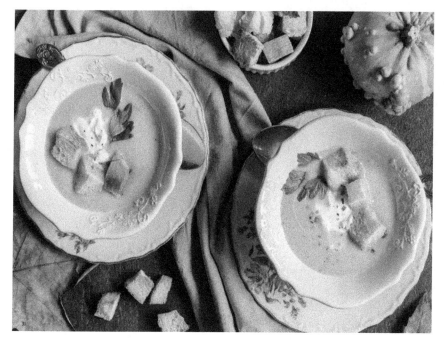

Servings Provided: 2-3

Time Required: 25 minutes

What is Needed:

- Chicken stock (6 cups)
- Freshly minced lemongrass (4 tbsp.)
- Makrut lime leaves (3 left whole) or substitute Lime zest(1 tsp.)
- Shallot (1 minced) or Purple onion (.25 cup minced)
- Garlic (3 cloves)
- Galangal or ginger (1 thumb-size piece)
- Fresh red chili (1) or dried crushed chili (.25-.5 tsp.) or chili sauce (1-2

tsp.)

- Pumpkin/squash (3 cups)
- Sweet potato/yams (2 cups)
- Ground coriander (.75 tsp.)
- Turmeric (.5 tsp.)
- Ground cumin (1 tsp.)
- Fish sauce (2 to 3 tbsp./as desired)
- Shrimp paste (.5-1 tsp.) or fish sauce(1 extra tbsp.)
- Brown sugar (1 tsp.)
- Lime juice - fresh-squeezed (2 tbsp.)
- Thick coconut milk (1/3 to 1/2 can)
- Soft tofu (1 to 2 cups - sliced into cubes/substitute chickpeas or cooked shrimp)
- Baby spinach - washed (1 generous handful)
- Fresh basil - the topping (.5 cup)

Preparation Method:

1. Pour the stock into the pot to warm using the high-temperature setting.
2. Rinse the spinach.
3. Mince and add the lemongrass (the stalk too if it's fresh), garlic, shallot, the makrut lime leaves, galangal or ginger, and chili. Wait for it to boil.
4. Peel, dice, and mix in the squash and yam. Adjust the temperature setting slightly and gently boil for six to seven minutes.
5. Meanwhile, whisk the spices and stir well after each addition (ground coriander, turmeric, cumin, shrimp paste, fish sauce, lime juice, and brown sugar).
6. Once the pumpkin and yams are softened, adjust the temperature

174

setting to low. Fold in the coconut milk as desired.

7. Give it a taste test to adjust the seasonings to your liking.

8. Just before serving, gently mix in the spinach and softened tofu.

9. Serve and garnish it using the coriander and basil.

10. Enjoy it with a serving of noodles or rice.

Red Curry With Bamboo Shoots & Coconut Milk

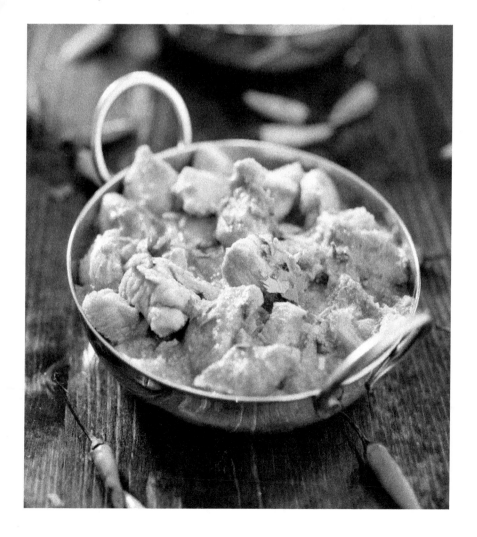

Servings Provided: 2

Time Required: 20 minutes

What is Needed:

- Boneless - skinless chicken thigh meat (1 lb./cut into ½-inch pieces)
- Coconut milk (2 cups - divided into two portions)
- Thai red curry paste (3 tbsp.)
- Bamboo shoots - canned or prepared - cut into thin strips (1 cup)
- Thai long chilies/another mild red chili (2-3)
- Thai sweet basil/Horapah-Star of Siam (1 cup)
- Kaffir lime leaves (5)
- Coconut Sugar (2 tsp.)
- Salt (.5 tsp./as needed)
- Fish Sauce (1 tbsp./as needed)

Preparation Method:

1. To get started, warm half the coconut milk in a wok or pan. Stir in the curry. Cook it using the low-temperature setting until it is thick and well blended.
2. Add the chicken stir-fry in the curry for about five minutes, and add the other half of the coconut milk.
3. Fold in the bamboo shoots, pieces of kaffir lime leaf, and red chilies. Simmer it for five minutes and let it cool.
4. Stir in the basil and serve

Chapter 2: Poultry

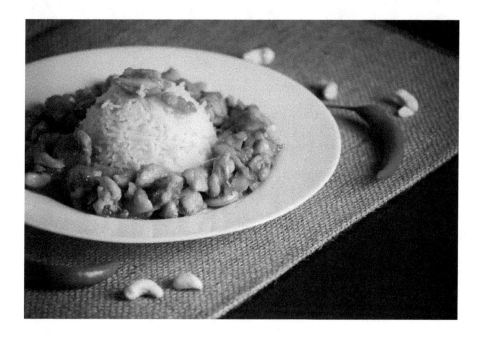

Cashew Chicken

Servings Provided: 2-4

Time Required: 20 minutes

What is Needed:

- Chicken legs - boneless & skinless (1 lb)
- Unsalted - raw cashew nuts (.5 cup)
- Thai long chilies (red & green/4-6)
- Wax peppers (1-2)

- Sun-dried Thai long chili (3-4)
- Brown/yellow onion (half of 1 small)
- Green onions (2-3)
- Garlic (2-3 large cloves)
- A-P flour (.25 cup)
- Finely cracked white pepper (.25 tsp.)
- Dark sweet soy sauce (.5 tsp.)
- Oyster sauce (2 tbsp.)
- Sugar (1 tsp.)
- Light soy sauce (.5 tsp.)
- For Frying: Vegetable Oil (1 cup)
- Water (.25 cup/as needed)

Preparation Method:

1. Dice the chicken into chunky pieces. Dice the onion, chilies, and green onions, and garlic.
2. Deep-fry the dried chilis, cashew nuts, and the chicken. Set them aside and dump the oil (reserving one tablespoon).
3. Sauté the garlic and onion. Mix in the sauces and sugar with a bit of water to make a gravy.
4. Fold in the fried chicken and stir until coated in the gravy. Simmer it for about two minutes.
5. Add the fried cashew nuts and simmer for a minute, and add the fresh chilies. Thoroughly mix and cook for 30 seconds.
6. Serve topped with the fried, dried chili pieces.

Chicken & Basil Stir-Fry

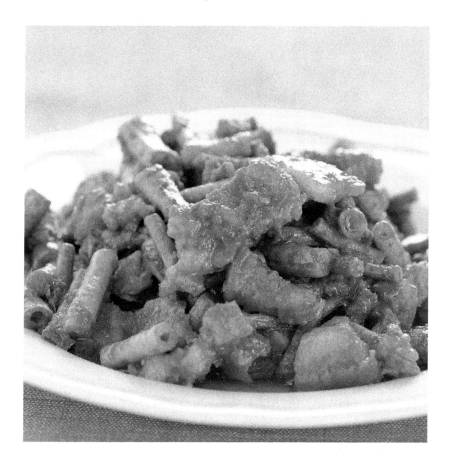

Servings Provided: 3-4

Time Required: minutes

What is Needed:

- Bone-in with skin chicken breast halves (1 lb.)

- Vegetable oil (1 tbsp.)

- Fresh ginger & garlic (1 tbsp. each)

- Hot chili flakes (.25 tsp.)

- Fat-skimmed chicken broth (2/3 cup)

- Soy/Asian fish sauce (1 tbsp.)

- Cornstarch (2 tsp.)

- Fresh basil leaves (3 cups - lightly packed)

- Salt

- Also Needed: Nonstick skillet (8-10-inch)

Preparation Method:

1. Mince the garlic and ginger.
2. Rinse and dab the chicken dry. Slice it crossways into strips 2-3 inches long and are about 1/8-inches thick.
3. Warm the skillet using the high-temperature setting and add the oil.
4. Toss in the chicken, chili flakes, ginger, and garlic.
5. Stir frequently and cook for about three to four minutes. (The pink in the center should be gone.
6. Whisk the cornstarch, fish sauce, and broth in a mixing container. Pour it into the pan and stir for about one minute.
7. Mix in the basil leaves, stirring about 30 seconds until they are wilted and dust with salt to serve.

Easy Thai Chicken

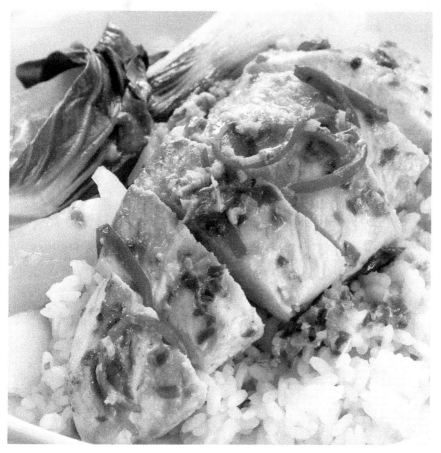

Servings Provided: 8

Time Required: 40 minutes

What is Needed:

- Unsalted butter (2 tbsp.)
- Peanuts (.25 cup)
- Cilantro leaves (2 tbsp.)
- Chicken thighs (8)

The Sauce:

- Sweet chili sauce (.5 cup)
- Soy sauce (2 tbsp.)
- Garlic (2 cloves)
- Fish sauce (1 tbsp.)
- Fresh ginger (1 tbsp.)
- Sriracha (1 tsp./as desired)
- Juice of 1 lime

Preparation Method:

1. Set the oven temperature at 400° Fahrenheit.
2. Chop the cilantro leaves and peanuts. Mince/grate the garlic and ginger.
3. Prepare the sauce by whisking the soy sauce, fish sauce, chili sauce, ginger, garlic, Sriracha, and lime juice in a mixing container and set it aside.
4. Prepare a large oven-proof skillet using the med-high temperature setting to melt the butter.
5. Add the chicken to the skillet and sear it (skin-side down) until golden brown (2-3 min. per side). Stir in chili sauce mixture.
6. Set a timer and roast until it reaches an internal temperature of 165° Fahrenheit (25-30 min.).
7. Switch it to the oven to broil to cook until caramelized and slightly charred (2-3 min.).
8. Serve them promptly topped with cilantro and peanuts.
9. Note: It's okay to leave the skin and bones on the chicken.

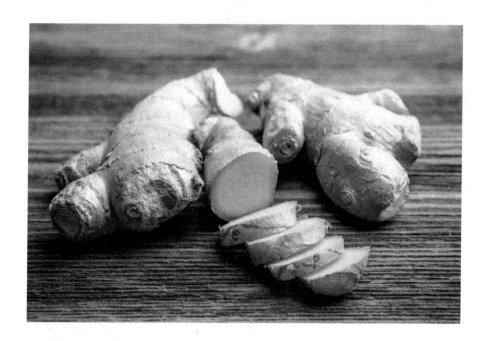

Ginger Chicken

Servings Provided: 2-4

Time Required: 20 minutes

What is Needed:

- Chicken breast (2 cups)
- Fresh ginger (1 cup)
- Cloud Ear Fungus (4 oz./about 100gm)
- Green onions (2 to garnish & 2 for the recipe/4 whole)
- Thai long chili/another mild red chili (2)
- Garlic (3-4 large cloves)
- Oyster sauce (2 tbsp.)

- Light soy sauce (2 tsp.)

- Palm/light brown sugar (1 tsp.)

- Black pepper (.5 tsp.)

- Vegetable oil (1 tbsp.)

Preparation Method:

1. Do the prep. Thinly slice the chicken. Peel and julienne the ginger and mince the garlic.

2. Sauté the garlic in the oil for about half a minute, and arrange the chicken in the skillet. Sauté it for about two minutes, stirring continuously.

3. When the chicken is almost done, add the sugar, black pepper, soy sauce, and oyster sauce. Stir and fry until the sugar melts, and the pan is sticky. Add a little water to make a thick sauce.

4. Add the Mouse Ear fungus and cook for another two minutes.

5. Fold in the ginger, green onion, and red chili.

6. Toss all of the fixings and continue to stir-fry for about one minute until it's all piping hot. Serve promptly.

Green Curry Chicken

Servings Provided: 4

Time Required: 28 minutes

What is Needed:

- Green curry paste (2 tbsp.)
- Fresh ginger (1 tbsp.)
- Light coconut milk (14 oz. can)
- Fish sauce (2 tsp.)
- Shredded dark meat chicken (.75 cup)
- Shredded chicken breast (.5 cup)
- Lime juice (1 tbsp.)
- Garlic clove (1 minced)
- Sesame oil (1 tbsp.)
- Sliced baby bok choy (3 cups)
- Sliced red bell pepper (1 cup)
- Uncooked wide brown rice noodles (5 oz.)
- Cilantro leaves (.5 cup)
- Lime (4 wedges)

Preparation Method:

1. Peel and grate the ginger. Combine the first four fixings (up to the line) in a saucepan using the medium-high temperature setting. Once boiling, adjust the setting to simmer for 15 minutes. Fold in the chicken

and simmer for another five minutes.

2. Transfer the pan to a cool burner and mix in the freshly-squeezed lime juice.

3. Warm oil in a skillet using the med-high temperature setting. Mix in the bok choy and bell pepper. Sauté them for two minutes and mix in the garlic. Continue to sauté them for 30 seconds.

4. Prepare the noodles per the package direction. Dump it into a colander to drain. Portion the noodles into four servings, topping each with ½ cup chicken mixture and ½ cup of the vegetables.

5. Garnish the chicken using the cilantro, and serve with a side of lime wedges.

Spicy & Salty Fried Chicken Wings

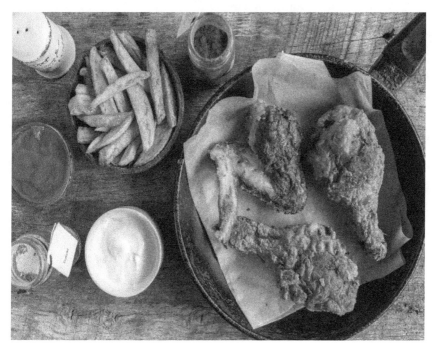

Servings Provided: 8-12

Time Required: 30 minutes

What is Needed:

- Chicken wings (3 lb.)
- Thai red curry paste (2 tbsp./as desired)
- Ground - dried Thai hot chili (1-2 tsp.)
- Oyster sauce (1 tbsp.)
- Sugar (1 tsp.)
- Fish sauce (1-2 tsp.)

- Water (.5 cup as needed)
- Optional Garnish: Kaffir lime leaves (6-8)
- Vegetable oil (.5 cup/as needed)

Preparation Method:

1. Whisk the fish sauce, oyster sauce, sugar, ground chili, and one tablespoon of red curry with the water.
2. Pour the mixture over the wings to marinate for a minimum of four hours.
3. Transfer the marinated chicken to a platter.
4. Mix in about one to two tablespoons of flour to the sauce and whisk it to create a thin batter.
5. Dust the chicken with flour, and dip them into the batter until they're well coated.
6. Deep fry them (in oil) for three to five minutes per side. Place them on a layer of paper towel towels to drain the excess fat.
7. Top with a portion of the crispy fried kaffir lime leaves.

Spicy Stir-Fried Chicken With Eggplant

Servings Provided: 2-4

Time Required: 10 minutes

What is Needed:

- Whole chicken leg (1 large - boneless & skinless)
- Thai eggplants (6-8)
- Thai long chilies/Mild green chiles (3-4)
- Thai sweet basil/leaves & flower tops (1 cup)
- Light soy sauce (2 tsp.)
- Sugar (.5 tsp.)
- Thai red curry paste (1.5-2 tbsp.)
- Fish sauce (2 tsp.)

Preparation Method:

1. Chop the chicken into bite-sized pieces. Pluck the leaves from the basil and cut the eggplant and chilis.
2. Fry the chicken with the red chili until thoroughly cooked. Add in the eggplant and continue cooking for about three to four minutes.
3. Mix in the mild green chili, and simmer it for another minute, and transfer the pan from the burner.
4. Garnish it using basil and enjoy the dish promptly.

Chapter 3: Beef

Basil Beef

Servings Provided: 4

Time Required: 30 minutes

What is Needed:

- Vegetable oil (2 tbsp.)
- Shallots (2)
- Garlic (7 cloves)
- Fresh ginger (1 tbsp.)
- Red bell pepper (half of 1)
- Lean ground beef (1 lb.)
- Brown sugar (2 tsp.)
- Soy sauce - low-sodium (6 tbsp.)
- Fish sauce (2 tbsp.)
- Asian garlic chili paste (2 tbsp./to taste)
- Oyster sauce (3 tsp.)
- Beef broth - low-sodium (.5 cup)
- Water (.25 cup)
- Cornstarch (1 tsp.)
- Basil leaves (1 cup)
- For Serving: Jasmine rice

Preparation Method:

1. Thinly slice the shallots and pepper. Mince the ginger and garlic. Set them aside.

2. Warm a large skillet/wok using the med-high temperature setting to heat the oil. When it's hot, toss in the peppers, ginger, garlic, and shallots to stir-fry for about three minutes.

3. Push the vegetables to the side and adjust the temperature setting to high. Add the beef, breaking it apart as it cooks.

4. Whisk the water, broth, cornstarch, chili paste, oyster sauce, fish sauce, soy sauce, and brown sugar. Simmer the sauce for about two minutes.

5. Toss in the basil and stir fry until it's wilted. Serve over cooked rice.

Steak Noodle Bowl

Servings Provided: 4

Time Required: 21 minutes

What is Needed:

- Green cabbage (2.5 cups)
- Freshly squeezed lime juice - divided (1 tbsp.)
- Kosher salt (1 tsp. - divided)
- Sugar (2 tsp. - divided)
- Uncooked flat-brown rice noodles - ex. Annie Chun's pad Thai-type (8 oz.)
- Top sirloin steak (12 oz.)
- Canola oil (1.5 tsp.)
- Water (.5 cup)

- Red curry paste - ex. Thai Kitchen (2 tbsp.)
- Light coconut milk (13.5 oz. can)
- Optional: Lime wedges (4)

Preparation Method:

1. Thinly slice the cabbage and add one teaspoon of juice, ½ teaspoon sugar, and ¼ teaspoon of salt. Toss and set it aside for about 15 minutes.
2. Prepare the noodles per the instructions provided on the package. Dump them into a colander to rinse and drain using fresh-cool water.
3. Toss the steak with about ½ teaspoon of sugar.
4. Prepare a skillet using the high-temperature setting to warm the oil.
5. Trim and slice the steak into thin strips and add it to the pan to simmer for about two minutes. Flip it over to cook for another half minute and remove it from the pan. Set it aside and keep it warm.
6. Add about ½ of a cup of water to the pan, scraping it to loosen browned bits. Add the curry paste and coconut milk, stirring well to combine. Wait for it to simmer.
7. Adjust the temperature setting to low and continue cooking for five minutes. Mix in the remaining two teaspoons lime juice, remaining one teaspoon sugar, and ½ teaspoon salt.
8. Arrange about one cup of the noodles in each of the four bowls and add the steak.
9. Ladle about ¼ cup of the broth over each serving and top each with about ½ cup of the cabbage mixture. Sprinkle the remaining ¼ teaspoon of salt evenly over each of the servings. Serve with lime wedges, if desired.

Chapter 4: Seafood

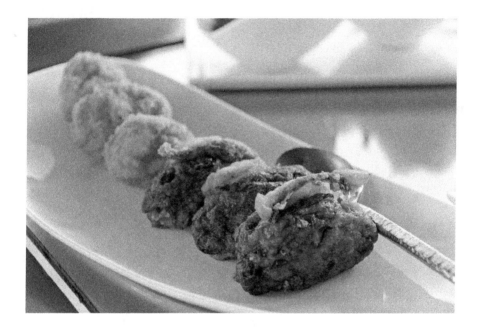

Thai Fish Cakes

Servings Provided: 20 small cakes

Time Required: 25 minutes

What is Needed:

- Whitefish fillets - cod or halibut (approx.13.5 oz.)
- Red curry paste (2 tbsp.)
- Green beans (.75 cup)
- Egg (1)

- Cornstarch (1 tbsp.)
- Sugar (1 tsp.)
- Fish sauce (1 tbsp.)
- Lime leaves (5)
- Vegetable oil (3 cups)

Preparation Method:

1. Chop the fish into small pieces and toss it into a food processor.
2. Break and add in the egg, cornstarch, curry paste, sugar, fish sauce, and blend until mixed. (*Don't puree* the mixture.)
3. Finely slice the green beans and lime leaves to combine with the mixture.
4. Form the mixture into patties, using about one tablespoon and shape until they are about two inches in diameter.
5. Add oil to a saucepan using the high-temperature setting and deep-fry the cakes.
6. Once the oil is sizzling, arrange the cakes in the saucepan and cook them until they are golden brown. Place the fish cakes onto a layer of paper towels to absorb the oil before serving.
7. Serve hot with sweet chili sauce (see the recipe below) with cucumber and crushed peanuts.

Sweet and Chili Sauce

What is Needed:

- Sugar (3 tbsp.)
- White vinegar (2 tbsp.)
- Salt (.25 tsp.)
- Water (2 tbsp.)
- Garlic (1 clove)
- Fresh chilies (2)
- Cucumber (2 tbsp.)
- Crushed peanuts (1 tbsp.)

Preparation Method:

1. Whisk the water, sugar, salt, and vinegar in a small mixing container. Pop it into the microwave for one minute.
2. Mince and add the garlic and chili in the bowl and thoroughly mix it.
3. Chop and add the cucumber and sprinkle with the peanuts.

Thai Green Curry With Seafood

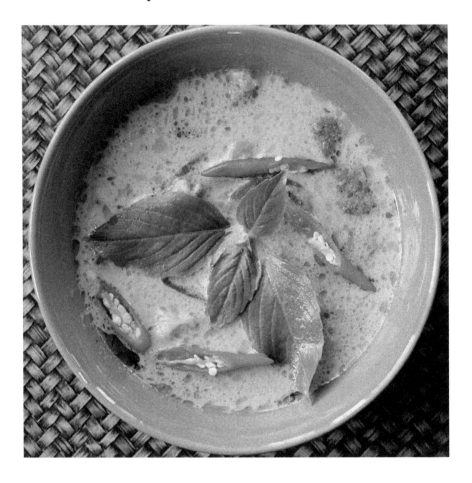

Servings Provided: 4

Time Required: 20 minutes

What is Needed:

- Unrefined peanut oil (2 tbsp.)

- Garlic cloves (3 minced)
- Green onions (5)
- Cilantro (3 tbsp. - divided)
- Thai green curry paste (6 tbsp.)
- Water (1.25 cups)
- Unsweetened coconut milk (13-14 oz. can)
- Kaffir lime leaves (2)
- Red jalapeño chile (1) OR Thai red chiles (2 small)
- Fish sauce - ex. nam pla or nuoc nam (1 tbsp.)
- Carrot (1 large/about 1 cup)
- Bok choy (4 cups)
- Uncooked medium shrimp (8 oz.)
- Bay scallops (8 oz.)
- Green or black mussels (1 lb.)
- Fresh basil (2 tbsp.)
- Steamed rice (2 cups)

Preparation Method:

1. Do the prep. Finely chop the dark green parts of the onion - separated from white and pale green parts. Mince the cilantro, garlic, basil, and onion.
2. Peel and thinly slice the carrot and bok choy. Peel and devein the shrimp. Scrub and debeard the mussels.
3. Prepare a large saucepan using the medium-temperature setting to warm the oil. Add the white and pale green parts of green onions, garlic, and one tablespoon cilantro. Sauté them until tender (2 min.)

4. Add the curry paste, sautéing it for about one minute until it's fragrant.

5. Add coconut milk, water, lime leaves, chilies, and fish sauce. Once it's simmering, add the carrots and cover. Cook until the carrot is tender (5 min.).

6. Layer the bok choy, scallops, mussels, and shrimp in the pan. Cover and simmer them until the seafood and bok choy are cooked, and the mussels have opened. Discard any of the mussels that do not open after about five minutes.

7. Stir in two tablespoons of the cilantro, the dark green parts of green onions, and basil.

8. Portion rice among four shallow bowls. Ladle the curry over rice and serve.

Thai Grilled - Baked Fish

Servings Provided: 4-6

Time Required: 1 ¼ hours – varies

What is Needed:

- Frozen whole milkfish (1 @ 2.5-3.5 lb.)
- Sea salt (1.5 tbsp.)
- Oyster sauce (1/3 cup)
- Thai soy sauce (2 tbsp.)
- Sugar (.5 tsp.)
- Fresh lemongrass (1 piece - smashed)
- Chef's knife (For cleaning the fish)

Preparation Method:

1. Thaw the fish overnight in the fridge. Thoroughly rinse it using cool water.
2. Use the knife to make three gashes on each side of the fish. Cover the fish with sea salt and let it rest for ten minutes.
3. Set the oven temperature at 350° Fahrenheit.
4. Place the fish into a large sheet of heavy-duty foil.
5. Combine the soy sauce, oyster sauce, and sugar. Dump it over the top of the fish and wrap it, crimping the edges of the foil on top to seal it shut.
6. Bake them for 40 minutes. You can also choose to grill over hot coals

for 50 minutes.

7. Check for doneness by flaking the flesh with a fork. When it's fully cooked, the meat should be flaky and white, not opaque. Leave the fish in the foil - undisturbed - for ten minutes.

8. Serve in the foil, on top of a large platter of red or green leaf kale or lettuce. Serve with a serving of jasmine rice (see the recipe).

9. Note: How to Clean the Fish: Scale the fish outside near a water source. Hold the knife at a 30-degree angle, scraping the scales away from yourself. Make a 3-inch incision at the stomach area, near the bottom edge of the fish. Trash the guts and leave the head and fin intact (if desired). You can skip all of this and purchase the fish pre-cut in the market.